HOW TO TRICK YOURSELF INTO FEELING YOUR FEELINGS

HOW TO TRICK YOURSELF INTO FEELING YOUR FEELINGS

Even After Decades of Numbness and Trauma

VERA WILHELMSEN

I published this myself :)

May you find the tools to heal
May you be brave enough to go inwards
May you heal so much that you can be in your body again
May you know what true relaxation means
May you find the courage to be yourself no matter what,
and there find the highway to happiness
May you build a life based on who you truly are and what you
truly want
May you learn to be proud of yourself and to love yourself
May you know inner peace
May you know safety
May you learn to take care of yourself as well as you take care of
your cat :)
A-friggin-men!

- Vera Wilhelmsen

I have written and rewritten this trigger warning and disclaimer many times. In my experience therapy and healthcare has been extremely toxic and deficient and I had to figure out how to heal from both chronic illness and trauma on my own. It therefore feels disgusting to write a disclaimer saying I'm not a licensed medical professional and that they know better - because they don't always. I will however say that I really am not a licensed medical professional and my claims have not been tested systematically on other people. Everything in this book is my own experience and my own opinions. I cannot guarantee any results or the safety of these tools. Use this book with caution, listen to your body and your feelings, and reach out for professional help if you need to.

Everything in this book is also very triggering. I believe avoidance keeps us stuck in endless loops and small lives, and that triggers can be healed with the right tools in place. However, you know yourself best, and it is up to you to discern whether it is safe for you to proceed and when it is time to take a break or stop altogether.

The first chapter is my story, which is a dark one, but also one of triumph. If you feel emotions coming up while reading my story, try pausing and writing down how you feel in a journal or on a piece of paper. Maybe suppressed feelings of hopelessness, frustration, anger or grief need your love and attention? And if it makes you angry that I am telling my story, know that you are not a bad person and I do not hold it against you. Ask yourself in what ways have you been silenced? You can turn to the "Instant Relief"-chapter at any time should the need arise, where you will find tools you can implement right away. You are also welcome to read this book in any order that feels good to you, or even skip entire chapters if that is what you need to do right now. Thank you for being here, thank you for making the world a better place by working on yourself and thank you for honoring my story!

Best of luck!

Vera

CONTENTS

CHAPTER 1

My Story

Hello, brave person! I am so grateful and honored that you would like to test-read a few pages and find out if this girl can actually help you ;) I believe I can! But before we get started, let me share a little bit about myself.

I'm Vera, an almost-thirty-year-old woman from Norway and my sign is Leo! I collect cute candy wrappers and shells and my vibe is "cute but will fight you." There is nothing I treasure more than colors, joy and happiness - and I don't allow anyone to rain on my parade! Throughout the following pages you will come to understand why I treasure the little things in life and why I protect myself with fierce boundaries. A few years ago, writing this book and expressing myself so honestly as I am going to in the following pages, would have been impossible. I used to be terrified of journaling, sending messages and emails, or having *any* sort of written or recorded evidence from *me*. I believed that anything written or recorded would somehow be found later and become evidence proving how bad and perverted of a person I was. I even believed I was unknowingly a criminal; that I somehow was walking around, doing horrible, illegal stuff without knowing it. You might have guessed it already: I grew up with a narcissistic mother. Scratch that, I *survived* and grew into adulthood in spite of my narcissistic mother. And father. And grandparents. And aunts. And uncles.

Everything I said was always wrong and mocked into oblivion. If I told a joke all the adults around me would start yelling. Were my jokes really that bad? Or did they have a horrible double meaning I didn't understand? I deeply believed that all my social instincts were damaged because how else could *everything* I said be wrong and *everyone* thought so? *No one in my family liked me.* What do you think that does to a child? Let's just say it didn't do wonders for my confidence or my will to live. I truly believed there was something wrong with me and that I was ugly, stupid and every other negative word in the dictionary. I lost trust in all of my feelings and instincts, as everything I said was mocked or ended up with me getting yelled at for being selfish and bad.

Turns out my inner compass wasn't broken. I was just trapped with people who felt better when they made children feel horrible about themselves. I come from a severely dysfunctional and abusive family where mistreatment, rejection and bullying has been passed down harder than DNA. (Look at me writing so *clearly* and with absolutely no sugar-coating! Hell yeah!) As a child I always had the feeling that my parents, aunts, uncles and grandparents wanted to kill me. Every day they filled me up with pain that would make any child wish for death. One day of this pain would be enough to want to commit suicide, and I experienced thousands of them. I had this feeling my family were trying to kill me without getting their hands dirty. They would push me to suicide instead. And as you will find out later in my story, they almost succeeded twice. But here I am, happy, gorgeous, intelligent and healthy, finally telling the truth and what I have learned from all of this. I have alchemized my pain into a beautiful life, art and helpful tools for others, while they are still running around in the same patterns. In my "family" children are abused, rejected and mistreated by their parents, and grow up to do the same thing to their children without thinking - and around and around we go. It's a cycle of shit! Well, until I came along! I often wonder if there was anyone else in my lineage, before my time, who felt the same way that I do, who saw the dysfunction and felt it in their hearts how wrong it is - and broke out of it or perished from it. Probably never to be mentioned again. *Secrets,* aka *truth,* is buried in toxic families. Any individual who leaves the family is deemed "crazy" and never spoken of again, pretended out of existence. Toxic families function like cults. If toxic relationships go on for long enough it usually goes one of these two ways - dying or breaking out. There is no inbetween. At some point you have to make a choice if you want to *live* or not. I have been close to death twice, first from a suicide attempt, the second time from getting very physically ill due to decades of unrelenting stress. Never think that it's "not that bad." Poison will kill you even in small doses if you take it every day. Value your nervous system and don't let toxic people impact it. Domestic violence isn't only physical. Don't let anyone tell you that emotional abuse isn't *real,* or isn't abuse. It is.There isn't only sexual and physical abuse in this world. And those two come *with* emotional and psychological abuse. It is all connected in one big shitshow. Emotional, psychological and verbal abuse kills slowly and sneakily. It was after almost three decades of abuse behind closed doors I realized that staying meant death, and I found the strength to break out. The unknown was suddenly less scary and less threatening than the known - and I was ready to make a move!

I CHANGED MYSELF

I've been looking for answers to "solve" my family situation since as early as I can remember. I can remember the moment I came to the conclusion that crying is bad and expressing my emotions doesn't work. I was maybe 3 years old, at least I was shorter than the sofa table as I was standing right next to it. I was crying loudly, and my mom yelled at me for doing so. She made me feel like I had done something horrible. She looked angry and afraid. I stopped crying and came to an internal conclusion that crying loudly or expressing anything wasn't safe and did not lead to anything good. I began changing myself and choosing my words with extreme caution already from the age of three. Extreme post traumatic stress disorder (PTSD) and exhaustion built up over the next twelve years until I was sixteen years old. I had exhausted all options I knew that could make my parents happy, or at least treat me better. I let my mom decide all of my clothing. I was quiet most of the time to not annoy them; I stayed in my room as much as possible to not be "in the way." I was doing my best in school to avoid criticism or to make them look like the bad parents they really were, to teachers and my classmates' parents (public image is more important to abusive parents than the health and wellbeing of their children.) I played the cello three times a week and during the weekends - and *nothing* made them proud or happy, or at least kick back 10% of the abuse. So I stopped eating. This decision came to be from exhaustion, desperation and the simple fact that it was the only thing I could think of that I had yet to try. Pleasing them and changing myself in their image hadn't worked, and of course all thoughts of protest had been beaten and scared out of me before I turned five - so what else could

I do other than refuse to live? I basically went on strike. I couldn't go on any longer. And I knew in my heart I wouldn't survive three more years of this until I turned 19, when I would finish high school and be able to move out. I knew I wouldn't last that long, so not eating was my last attempt of survival and change - *any* change.

So, not eating eventually ended me up in child therapy, or BUP (department for child- and youth psychiatry in Norway.) Not because my parents were worried (my mother yelled at me for daring to annoy her with an eating disorder), but because my best friend went to the school nurse. My silent plea was heard. Or so I thought... I entered into a three year long nightmare of circular conversations where the therapists would avoid any real and deep conversation and emotions like the plague. I carefully tried to explain the sneaky ways of my parents' abuse. This was extremely hard and I was terrified it would get me into more trouble. But all I was met with was a broken record of "she probably didn't mean it that way," "you live in Norway, we have free school here, you are a lucky child," "your parents have higher education, only parents without education abuse their children" and my favorite: "you're one of those *good girls* aren't you? You just put too much pressure on yourself in school - that's why you're depressed." *Depressed?* If you want to call being close to death from sixteen years of relentless abuse being depressed, then maybe you should consider a career change. Why wasn't I allowed to call a spade a spade? To just say *exactly* what I felt. To feel the relief of truth and authentic expression. "You ruminate too much," they told me. I was sixteen years old, it was impossible that there was anything wrong with my psyche that didn't come from my environment and that you, the "professional," it is your job to help me with this rumination, not tell me it's my fault and I should "just stop." Children aren't responsible for their actions or their psyches in the same way adults are, all guidance has to come from their environment.

SOMETHING "WRONG" WITH THE CHILD = SOME-
THING WRONG WITH THE CHILD'S ENVIRON-
MENT AND THE PEOPLE AROUND THE CHILD,
NOT THE CHILD ITSELF.

- Vera wilhelmsen, self-quoter and someone who is
finally speaking up

I mean, six years at university and that's the best you could do? Why were we going around in circles about "automatic thoughts," rumination and everything *I* had to do to change *me*, because all my troubles were my own fault from "putting too much pressure on myself" and being a "good girl." Writing this makes me want to puke and punch something. I have a high risk of going off on a tangent here, but the term *good girl* has somehow become a way of blaming teenagers for their problems when it's clearly the adult world that has created the horrible environments the teenagers react to. Anyway, it made no sense to spend all of this time on shallow "treatments" while I was not provided with help to find the words to express the deep pain and grief of what was going on at home, and most importantly: HELP WITH GETTING OUT OF THERE. I should have been rescued from that house of horrors the day I was born. But there I was sixteen years later, surrounded by professionals, in "the world's best healthcare system" in "the best country in the world" (only Norwegians say this), and receiving *no help*. It wasn't just no help, they were making it worse! A lot worse. My self-blame and shame increased in therapy. All I needed was to be validated, to express my pain, to be heard and to be removed out of abuse. Is that really too much to ask of people who've studied the human psyche for at least six years? Is it too much to ask of someone to make a twenty minute call to child-protection services? Apparently it is. That's why I'm writing this book. So *you* can have access to this fundamental information which for some reason is so hard to come by. I had to almost *die* to find this information, I mean WHAT THE FRICK. I had to do deep digging on the internet and do countless experiments on myself to *invent* the healing methods shared in this book, when this should be the *first thing* you hear about at any therapist's office and the first thing any future therapist should learn in school. Also, they should all go on an inner journey, process their own childhoods and see themselves clearly before they even *think* about touching another human's psyche. I don't believe that any of our thoughts or feelings are to be ignored or suppressed. We cannot outsmart any of it. The quickest way to "make it go away" is to go into it so deep that it feels heard, seen and becomes healed. Then you don't have to ignore "bad" or painful thoughts anymore, because they won't be there when there's no *need* for them to beg for your attention anymore. *There's nothing wrong with your brain!* The thoughts and feelings come from *somewhere*, from trauma or conditioning/programming from family and society. SO FRIGGIN DO THE WORK THERE! At the *root*! Sorry, I wasn't shouting at you, but at all the toxic therapists of the world :) Candace van Dell said in one of her YouTube-videos that we live in an emotional dark-age, and I couldn't agree more.

The story of the world's biggest emotional circus at BUP continued as they set up the shitshow musical of *family therapy with two abusive parents*. Yeah. Take a moment to imagine how that went. Not good? Ding ding ding! You're absolutely correct! It mainly consisted of me struggling and exhausting myself for an hour trying to explain to *adults* how their behavior, their choice of words, their intention behind the words and how they make someone feel matters. They all laughed – yes, also the therapist – and explained away my concerns with "you will understand when you're older." Well, now

I'm 29 and I will sure as FECK never speak to any child or adult the way you spoke to me and I will never let any child in my care spend time with any toxic adults or "professionals" such as you. FECK. YOU. I mean, you can't just claim a get-out-of-jail-free-card by hiding your abuse in a mixed word-salad with a dressing consisting of "it's your fault." This was extremely hard to put into words, so I said things like "you're always so negative! You say things like love fades," I blurted out, while feeling the deep frustration and grief of trying to put words to their insane behavior and trying to explain it back to them, only to have it pushed aside with even more craziness and confusing "explanations" and "excuses." The therapist and my parents all laughed at me. I felt like I was drowning, not knowing if love and respect even existed and if I would ever be treated in a way that would make me feel good, when even professionals backed my parents' insanity as "normal." I've experienced firsthand how our society, including our school systems, government, healthcare systems and even therapy is very disconnected from love and truth.

This resulted in these questions running through my mind at sixteen years old:

- So I just have to adjust to bullying and insanity and fake, insane psychological environments. It's normal and I should just accept it?

- Since everyone is doing it it must be alright?

- Am I expecting too much?

- Am I ungrateful? My mother always says so...

- Am I too sensitive?

- Is everyone okay with this except me?

- Do I have to choose between isolation and pain?

- Does this mean that to be able to have a relationship with anyone you must take abuse on the chin and pretend it isn't there?

- Is it really impossible to create a clean, happy relationship?

My head was spinning. I was sixteen years old, exhausted from sixteen years of this craziness and now they were saying that I would have to endure this shit *for the rest of my life*. Just so you know: it doesn't have to be like this. Phew! Only with the wrong people. There are plenty of good, stable, healthy people out there you can have happy, chill, fun, belly-laugh-and-cuddle good times with! "All" you have to do is set new standards for who you allow into your life and stay strong in the inbetween-phase where you've broken up with all toxic people and you find yourself very temporarily alone! I don't think anyone should stay in relationships that are "only a little bit abusive" or "a little bit toxic." If there's a little bit of cyanide in the water, then the whole fish tank is poisoned. Yes, you are the fish in this example. You deserve clean water. No, you deserve the freedom of the open ocean or a beautiful coral reef depending on your preferences, and with the companionship of a lovely fish-friend if you want! I want to inspire you to break out of *all* toxic relationships, even the ones that aren't *that bad*. **A little bit of poison is too much poison.** It's unnecessarily draining and it holds you back in life. Imagine what you could do with all that energy you spend walking on eggshells and attempting to predict a toxic person's next moves! You could paint the new Sistine Chapel! You could live in a cabin in the woods! You could cure cancer! You could enjoy life! You could write a book! Like I'm doing now! It's because I have access to *all* my energy now that I'm not constantly being criticized every day that I am able to write this book! Life-changing! Walking on eggshells, constant criticism, constantly defending yourself, constantly playing small and constantly trying to predict what will upset the toxic person next is draining you more than you think. You're probably exhausted but since you're so used to it you don't realize how much more energy other people who aren't in toxic relationships have! They have *a lot more time and energy*! Looking back, my toxic family drained 98% of my energy on bullshit and I had 2% energy left to function in life. Functioning was hard.

Now let's talk about giving people consequences for their actions. If you're thinking "my mother has neglected me and said horrible things to me but I know deep down she loves me," maybe it's time your mother gets some appropriate consequences for her actions so she can make the choice to either *step up* or *step out* of your life. Raise your standards and let those who can't follow fall off. They have their own journeys to go on. You don't have to personally carry them through their irresponsible lives. When you touch a hot burner you will feel pain, pull your hand back, and *learn* that you shouldn't put your hands on hot burners. But when you stay in toxic relationships you magically take away the heat and pain from the toxic person's hand, preventing them from experiencing their *appropriate consequences*. They deserve people shouting "what the FECK, don't speak to me again!" back to them when they utter their stupid poison, not the enabling you're doing! They *need* to lose the people they mistreat, they *need* to feel the pain of their self-created isolations so that *maybe* they'll one day do better and do the healing work. Don't enable their *stuckness* while sacrificing yourself! Don't hold your breath and wait for toxic people to change - give them appropriate consequences, leave and *maybe* get back in touch *if* they've done *thorough* healing work. If you want to. Completely up to you. But take heed - it might be going okay for you *now*, staying in that toxic ass relationship that isn't "that bad," but I promise you it will be easier to leave *now* rather than a few more years down the line when you're even more damaged, mentally and physically, and you've lost *even more time* to stupid, uneccessary, draining bullshit. *Please leave!*

Just a heads up: the next part of the story is the heaviest part. Major trigger warning regarding self-harm and suicide! Please take care of yourself and journal through it if this brings up something in you, or skip it if you feel like that would be best for you right now.

THE FIRST DARK NIGHT OF THE SOUL

I ended up attempting suicide under the care of these "professionals" at BUP. It happened while I was staying in one of their facilities for a couple of weeks when I could not promise that I would be alive for the next session. This was around a month into my weekly sessions at the out-patient clinic, and I was sixteen years old. After I had been there for around a week I realized that the therapists at the facility had the same mindset as the ones at the clinic, and that they weren't going to help me out of the abuse. It makes me sick to this day remembering their smug faces as they shut me down, told me once again I was a *good girl* and felt like they'd done a good day's work. They repeated the unspoken rule that my purpose was to stroke the fragile egos of all adults I met, and that their feeling of doing a good job was more important than how I felt and if I even remained alive or not. I had noticed this unspoken rule at home, with grandparents, aunts and uncles and with the teachers at school.

Such NEGLECT! After a week they sent me on a two-day leave back home to my parents. As they picked me up they played the parts of concerned, loving parents, but as soon as the car-door shut they were quiet, and rage radiated from them. When we got home I was once again left alone in my room to contemplate how bad of a daughter I was and how I had *dared* to let nosy therapists into our "business." I cut my wrists on my bedroom floor. Not to die, but to get some relief from the shame and pain, and to maybe, just maybe, be taken seriously. My father walked in and said in a casual and mocking tone "aww, poor Vera," put a bandaid on the wound, gave me a couple of ironic pats on the back and left me there. He left me there. His child. This is for sure my worst memory of my father. His bottomless neglect and indifference was so apparent in this moment. As always I was left with my head and emotions spinning and no one to rely on to get me up off the floor than myself. I also cut myself in the emergency psychiatric facility. And they had the same response: casually putting a bandaid on it, acting like this was not a big deal and that this was everyday business for them. I remember they talked about the weather or something as they put a bandaid on my wrist, while internally I was reeling, trying to grasp their indifference and upside-down emotional world. A therapist even told me "what if in a few years you want to wear a dress and you can't because of your scars?" *That* was their therapy method for getting someone to stop self-harming. Stabilizing and stopping bad behaviors using shallow conversations, invalidation and motivating with shame and superficial stuff like wearing dresses... Modern therapy in a nutshell! Bleh. Not even starving yourself or cutting yourself got the attention, help or respect of all of these adults who had chosen to work in the children's mental health field. Why were they even there? And why is *seeing* someone and *validating* them so hard? Do they beat empathy out of future therapists during those six years at university? What the hell is going on? Out of pure desperation

I tried to choke myself with my own hands. I passed out and was found on the bathroom floor by one of the assistants at the BUP psychiatric emergency facility. She shook me and told me dinner was ready. And that was it. That. Was. It.

...

...

...

I have no words. It was never spoken of again. I didn't bring up the subject because I thought they ignored it, since I "hadn't done it properly" or "done it for attention." I thought they were ignoring what I had done to *shame* me. To this day this makes me want to puke and smash something. I wouldn't even wish the shame and confusion I felt on my abusers. Or... maybe I would. It was their shame to begin with. I wish I could go back in time and rescue little, beautiful sixteen year old Vera, get her the frick out of that insane psychological circus covering under the guise of "therapy" and "family," and tell her how she has *nothing* to be ashamed of! I would also tell her how she is perfectly normal while also being amazingly unique.

I was also drugged up on antidepressants and other toxins I don't even remember. I was given a sleeping pill in the psychiatric emergency care facility which made me extremely dizzy and drowsy for over 24 hours. I could barely sit up and keep my eyes open, and they shamed me for being lazy and for "not trying," and forced me to go out on a walk. How do they suddenly expect us to make our own decisions as adults when we are constantly overriden as children? I said I was too tired to take a walk, and they felt they knew better about my body. I was discharged from the emergency facility after two weeks, since a few days had gone by without me doing any more "dramatic" things, aka trying to choke myself and cut myself. That must mean I'was doing great, right? Had they secured a new living place for me, safe from my abusive parents? Nope. They all told me I was doing fine, so I guess it was true then? Nope. Once again adults had done a shitty, neglectful, shallow job and told me to be grateful for it. Everyone was always *telling me* how I was feeling and how I was doing. Back at the outpatient clinic where I went every week, they asked me every week if I "felt better," and every week I said "no" because *nothing had changed*, and every week they increased my dosage of antidepressants until I became bed bound at the age of seventeen with muscle spasms, a sleep that was more like coma, impossible to wake up from, and my sweat smelled like *paint*. They drugged me up and tried to numb my feelings away so they wouldn't have to do any *real* work, or simply *their job*. I also remember telling my main therapist that I was terrified of becoming like my parents if I didn't heal all the pain inside of me. He laughed and told me "we all end up like our parents anyway." Are. You. SERIOUS. In doing so he severely sabotaged and delayed my journey to healing said pain. I guess he ended up like his parents and took no responsibility for his behavior or impact on the unfortunate children in his care.

I have been told things have gotten a little better at BUP in the later years. But this wasn't even *that* long ago. I went there weekly from 2009 to 2011. If it has gotten better, it surely must vary from therapist to therapist. The *entire system* is in need of *serious* improvements. If this really is, which I doubt, *"the world's best healthcare system,"* then I am *terrified* for the rest of the world. Because what was done to me is a *joke*! A lethal one. I think a lot of therapists have blood on their hands due to their unconsciousness, ignorance and their own unresolved trauma. Again, we live in an emotional dark-age.

So after my suicide attempt and all of the increased shame, all I could do was clamp my jaw and try even harder to accept that abuse is just a part of society and every relationship, that I am just too sensitive and weak - and once again attempt to become a person that would make my parents love me. All my life they had looked down on all the *non-engineers* of the world, which is A LOT of people. I knew it was important to not be like all the groups of people they criticized to stay out of their line of fire, so I was going to become an engineer! In doing so I was hoping they would magically become different people, they would finally love me and I would finally have *real parents*! In the fall of 2013 I began a five year chemical engineering program called "Chemical Engineering and Biotechnology" at the Norwegian University of Science and Technology. Let's just say it didn't work out... Two and a half years into the study program I collapsed and didn't get up for three years. My stomach was constantly bloated and in pain, I had insomnia, nightmares and even sleep hallucinations. I woke up in panic attacks every morning. I gradually lost more and more function in my arms and legs. I walked with a serious limp and could not unclench my fists. I saw all the doctors, did all the tests and suffered through all the waiting in between. I freaked out as the finish line of graduation was pushed further and further into the future. At the time I believed getting the degree was my only hope of ever making my life better. I wondered if I could go back to school in a wheelchair. I tried to push myself back in school at all costs! And now I will present to you my experience in the *physical* health care system. Get ready for the next part of the shitshow musical! It gets worse before it gets better!

THE SECOND DARK NIGHT OF THE SOUL

I really believed I would be treated better in the physical health-care system as it would be based on facts and science and not the current collective mindset of the mental healthcare system - or the random mindset of your randomly assigned therapist. And since something was *physically* wrong then they must take it seriously and not stop until it's fixed, right? If I have *physical* ailments they must take it seriously, right? They wouldn't leave me in pain, would they? So naive... It turns out, you are at the mercy of your doctor's mindset here as well. And the physical healthcare system also has a collective mindset which has changed a lot over the years. So why is this one the correct one? Is this one *really* perfect? All I got out of the count-less hours in doctor's offices was a lot of "the blood tests don't show anything wrong," "I see you can't walk or use your hands but these tests don't *prove* what I'm seeing and what you're saying, which means it's all in your head and I don't care if you run a marathon to-morrow." Yes, a *neurologist* who clearly saw I was struggling to walk and had lost all function in my fingers told me "I don't care if you run a marathon tomorrow" because the *tests* didn't *prove* anything. So your job puts you under no obligation to help people without tests? And do you really think the tests we have measure everything in the body? If so, that is extremely arrogant and naive. I think we're only able to measure a tiny percentage of all bodily functions. When did doctors become pill-, surgery- and cream-dispensers instead of *healers*? When did doctors stop trying to get to the root of people's ailments and try to help them instead of gaslighting patients into believing that they are making it up for attention when their limited range of tests come back negative? And when the tests do come back positive, shouldn't we also work on reducing stress, removing toxic relationships, and finding true happiness instead of only doing pills and surgery? Why have we split illness into positive test = real and negative test = patient made it up for attention. And so what if your physical ailments disappear after you remove toxic relationships? The physical ailments were still real even though the causes were psychological stress. It's time to end the split between mental and physical health, and the stigma around mental health affecting our physical health. Now, I'm not gonna start another rant similar to the one about BUP, but let's just say that the physical healthcare system was just as big of a shitshow as the mental healthcare system... The only system I haven't tested yet is the *legal* system. And I don't plan on it as my confidence in it is extremely low after experiencing the other dysfunctional, unconscious, inhumane systems. That's why I chose not to go to court against my parents/abusers. I chose to do the healing work, become myself and share my story instead. And make money from joyful activities that make the world a better place, such as this book, instead of trying to make money from being chewed up and spat out in court. In all honesty I don't think building my life on compensation-money (if I even were to get it) from the abuse would have felt good. I chose to walk the path I deep down always wanted instead: find the answers to my healing and true emotional intelligence, and then become a writer and a filmmaker. I now share what I have learned and express my creativity on Instagram, on YouTube and in this book. Cheers to the first book of many! Starting a business was very triggering and I was forced to heal even more trauma and limiting beliefs such as "I need permission," "I'm not allowed" and "everything I do is bad and probably criminal, someone will come and get me." It was, and still is, a bumpy road, but I know I chose the right path as I have never breathed more deeply or felt more fulfilled! I have connected with people all over the world and received a lot of lovely emails from people telling me I have helped them. Thank you!

Aaaand back to my life story: so there I was, in my early twenties, supposed to be in my prime, unable to walk or use my hands, having gone through everything the healthcare system had to offer. There were no more doctors I could see and my general practitioner told me I "wasn't sick enough" to get a therapist. Once again they spat in my face. I *was* very sick, hanging on to life by a thread, both physically and mentally/emotionally. *I know*, it's infuriating! My hands and feet had stopped working from stress, but I didn't figure that out until *after* I had climbed out of this state and watched these symptoms temporarily come back only around my parents. It was terrifying to go through these symptoms and on top of it get no response or help from doctors. I truly believed I would die of some super-rare neurological condition while no one cared and no one would lose their medical license afterwards. I saw myself dying and there not even being an investigation following my death! No one would even blink over my death and the world would just keep spinning like I'd never existed. No consequences for all the people who abused and neglected me or for the medical neglect. It was a horrible thing to go through. Only people who haven't tested these systems believe they work and are amazing. I think to myself "oh, I hope you never have to find out!" and say nothing whenever the topic arises.

So there I was, waiting three months between every specialist doctor's appointment, beginning to realize that no one was coming to help me and provide a quick-fix that would put me back in school ASAP. I began looking for answers in other places and for ways to distract myself from the stress and pass the time. This was around the time the first *konmari* wave hit the world.

Konmari is a Japanese decluttering and tidying method created by Marie Kondo, meant not only to give you a tidier house, but to help you find out what is important to you, what brings *you* joy and to basically begin living this new life with less clutter and a more streamlined home. Pretty cool if you ask me! I began noticing that I felt very sad and overwhelmed every time I opened up my closet, which was crammed and filled with fast fashion in a style meant to avoid criticism from my mother. I dressed like her in light blue button-up shirts and navy cardigans. We have completely different complexions, and light blue and navy washes me out. And not to forget, I was in my early twenties and not a fifty-something professional! Where was the *color*, where was the *sexy* and fun clothing?? I dressed like a CEO of some boring, outdated, destroying-the-world-for-profit oil company when deep down I wanted to be a walking, sexy rainbow! Nothing wrong with classy clothing, but it wasn't my style or my choice.

I always felt like I had nothing to wear and I felt guilty about all the money I had spent on cheap dresses, and the environmental impact I was responsible for. My life felt completely out of my control and my closet felt like the right place to start gaining that control. So, I dragged my butt to a bookstore even though I felt like shit, and picked out my very own *The Life Changing Magic of Tidying Up* by Marie Kondo from a huge pile of pink books in the middle of the store. I was wearing my *navy* responsible-looking coat and dragging my numb feet after me. From the first pages I was *hooked*. I remember thinking "this is what *I* want! I've been looking for this but I couldn't put it into words," as I was reading about a woman who just *loved* mushrooms, they made her *so* happy, and after she had decluttered her home she put her entire mushroom-knick-knack collection on display so she could see them every day! During this time in my life I believed I was going to die, and my main motivation for decluttering my things was to throw out anything that my mother could use to talk shit about me after my death, such as anything in writing or any "shameful" panties. (I now own a drawer full of "shameful" panties, because I'm not an emotionally blocked baby-boomer who shames other people instead of working through their own pain, and healing your sexuality is an important part of the healing journey, you're welcome, thank you very much!) But this mushroom-lady sparked something in me! Maybe it was hope. Maybe it was permission to try to make yourself happy and the permission to adopt the perspective that your home is *your* place, it is there for *you*, it should be functional and work for *you* and you can do whatever you want with it! It makes me so happy writing this five years later, as I am healthy and strong. I went for a run yesterday and just finished putting together a glass cabinet displaying all my favorite things. It's filled with a distinct aesthetic, *my style*, and things that make me happy, such as high heels with glitter, Barbie furniture I found second hand, my camera to inspire me to keep pursuing filmmaking and my favorite books! The cabinet looks like my personal art installation, or what it looks like inside of my brain now that I have found myself! It's an external display of my inner world and what I value in life. It is *so me*!

So what the mushroom-lady had that I wanted was in essence: knowing your style (knowing yourself) and living by it. Marie Kondo would have my full blessing if she ever decides to change her motto from "the life-changing magic of tidying up" to "the life-*saving* magic of tidying up!" I couldn't have put it into words back then, but as this process unfolded, the konmari process revealed to me that my mind and heart were frazzled and in pieces. I had no idea how to make my own decisions, had no idea what my style was or what I wanted in *any* aspect of life, and most importantly: *I had never asked myself* what I wanted or liked. This really got me wondering: Why? Was my inner compass broken? Was I a boring person? Was I brain-damaged? (I seriously wondered about this often) Was I *born broken*, without any wants, likes or dislikes that made me distinguishable from other people? I felt like a gray blob always molding myself to accommodate everyone's wishes, whims, styles and opinions. Changing every day while dying on the inside. It would take me a few more years to figure all of this out, but I had become this way to keep myself as safe as possible. *To minimize pain.* My life with my abusive parents was extremely painful, but less painful when I let my mom make all my decisions, like controlling all my clothing indirectly, as I never bought anything that would upset her, which resulted in me dressing like a mini-version of her and avoiding any fun or criticism-worthy decorative pieces for my room, past-times, hobbies and friends. But she was still able to find fault in everything. Later I realized it wasn't about me, what I wore or what I did. She *wanted* and *needed* to criticize and upset me because of her own unresolved trauma and lack of self-responsibility.

I kept decluttering over the next two years. I got rid of everything that didn't *spark joy*, which was basically everything. All I have left from before I turned twenty-seven is a box with cupcakes on the exterior and my pokemon cards. I kid you not. Haha. And in all that *space* I began the journey of finding out what I like, and essentially *who I am.* I had to figure out how to build up a gut feeling that had been nuked, how to find my style when my brain was nothing but scrambled eggs and what the frick I wanted to fill my time with now that I had removed everything that wasn't me, even quitting school and putting down the cello. Maybe one day I will feel like playing again. For myself. I had never even been allowed to think about what I wanted for a career and I had no idea that free time existed for hobbies that *you* have chosen and that make *you* happy, and not for hobbies that make you *acceptable* to others. Not a single minute out of any given day was spent on my happiness or joy. I played the cello to please my unpleasable father and make my parents look good. I exercised to have an "acceptable" body and to not be judged as lazy, not because it felt good or was fun. My entire life was controlled by and lived for my parents. No wonder I felt dead inside! Luckily, because of my perseverance and willingness to try new things, the way I lived my life was *shifting* during this period. And the decluttering was extremely important in this shift.

Since I was now more conscious of what was lacking, what wasn't working in my life and what I needed going forwards, I was more open to new things. I read a lot of books and began journaling and writing down what my dream life would look like. More accurately, I *listened* to a lot of books while I spent 99% of my days in bed waiting for the next doctor's appointment in three months. I listened to a lot of books about intentional living and minimalism. Cortney Carver's content and book *Soulful Simplicity*, on simplifying her life and how it led to improvements with her chronic illness gave me hope. Finding myself was my sidequest while I trotted through the healthcare system, but it ended up being the main quest that healed me.

In 2018, there were no more doctors I could see. I had been spat out by the healthcare system. They had completely dropped me and there were no follow-ups or check ups while I was starving in a bed in my parent's home. The specialists had referred me to a "complex symptoms/illness" department which meant no more tests and a more psychosomatic approach. Having gone through the BUP shitshow I had very low hopes for this next step. I had already tried therapy and it had gotten me nowhere. I could also tell my mother was getting more and more agitated by the thought of someone once again "prodding in our business" and risking them finding out what was going on behind closed doors. She needed to keep the "*Vera is physically ill and I am such a wonderful mother taking care of her*"-story going as it gave her a lot of positive attention from colleagues. But it was not the truth. And the truth always comes out in the end. She is a sick child-abuser. And so is my father. His neglect and anger knows no bounds. They have not portrayed *any* parenting behavior and instead chosen to abuse. They did things they should not have done and did not do things they should have. There was a lack of the right things and a presence of the wrong things. You can suppress truth, but only temporary. Truth will erupt like a volcano. It is only a matter of time. And here we are.

TRUTH WILL ERUPT LIKE A VOLCANO. IT IS ONLY A
MATTER OF TIME.

- Vera Wilhelmsen, self-quoter and bearer of the name "Vera", which means "truth" in Latin origin. Suck on that, users and abusers.

I ended up canceling the psychosomatic appointment and went for a second opinion from a neurologist first, which my mother set up of course. The neurologist was of course of the same personality type as my mother, general practitioner and a lot of the specialist doctors. She acted like I was an annoying hypochondriac and sent me to a psychiatrist. This psychiatrist could have helped me if she had chosen a different approach than she did. She told me very bluntly that my relationship with my mother was very unhealthy. Claiming that our "relationship" was unhealthy insinuates I was a partaking, responsible party in this dynamic, which I was not. Be extremely careful about increasing guilt and shame in victims of abuse. She said it in a very judgmental, disciplining way. I told her I had already been to BUP and that they couldn't help me yada yada yada. She then yelled "can't you see this is unhealthy?!" Pro tip: try to understand the mind of someone who has been abused since birth or for an extended period of time. They are full of shame and confusion. They blame themselves and have been told repeatedly that the abusers have a right to treat them that way and that they are sensitive, stupid and dirty for feeling the way they feel. I was extremely ashamed of my inner pain, my symptoms and my inability to function. Telling me "you are not responsible for your mother," "no one has a right to talk to you the way your mother talks to you," "you have a right to make your own decisions," "not taking your feelings seriously is abuse" etc. would have been a lot more helpful. I was sent back to my general practitioner after this inconclusive "second opinion," with my head spinning. I asked my GP if she could send me to the psychosomatic department again and she straight up told me "no." I wish I felt powerful enough to change GPs at this time,but after meeting countless doctors with this personality type and mindset, I felt like there was no point and I felt like I would break if I went through one more session of invalidation and ridicule of my very real symptoms. I just couldn't do it anymore. Over two years of endless cycles of waiting, hoping, being ridiculed - repeat. She just said no. And she didn't provide any alternative plan. She would not send me to a therapist or the psychosomatic department because I wasn't "sick enough". I was 26, unable to walk, unable to use my hands and spent 99% of my time in bed avoiding sounds - and she couldn't care less. *Not sick enough*? Then what is? Being dead? I'm not sure if this is even legal. Aren't doctors bound by oath to help or something? Whatever, I am not spending another second of my life on that "doctor." I was lost. I was drowning. And she tied some extra stones to my feet.

After this fiasco there was nothing more for me in the healthcare system. No more doctors to see. All that was left was alternative therapies. I tried the keto diet, homeopathy, made tea from mushrooms that grow on dead trees, took lots of hot epsom salt baths and extreme amounts of expensive vitamins. I saw a private doctor who offered me low-dose-naltrexone to bypass the pain. I declined. I was *so* tired of symptom-management. I wanted a *cure* dammit! I wanted a doctor who could deep dive down to the root cause with me and help me do the work there. My frustration grew as my weight dwindled. In the fall of 2018 I was 40 kgs, had gray skin, gray lips, irregular heart rhythms, woke up every night feeling like I was choking, my eyes were burning and it felt like my kidneys were on fire. At this time I truly believed death was on my doorstep and I was running out of time. On Aileen Xu's podcast, *The Lavendaire Lifestyle,* about creating your best life I randomly came across a woman who also had experienced countless chronic symptoms and was now free of all of them. Her name was Sahara Rose Ketabi and she was talking about *Ayurveda*.

DON'T F*CK WITH ME

February 2019 I got a lot of my energy back pretty much overnight from doing an ayurvedic *panchakarma*. Ayurveda is the traditional health system of India, and a panchakarma is a gentle, rebalancing cleanse, consisting of gentle remedies such as eating rice, lentils and spices, taking herbs, receiving oil massages, steam therapy and rest. I was programmed to believe "alternative medicine" was for people who were too stupid to understand science, but since I had now realized how much stupidity and unconsciousness existed in society and that I didn't have to live my life however anyone told me - I was open to some new stuff. Ayurveda kickstarted my energy as it removed a lot of badly digested food by doing one day of fasting (nothing extreme like the seven day fasts we hear about), and eating meals I could actually digest and building up from there. At the time I was 40 kg and had been without appetite for many months. I am forever grateful for Ayurveda and for the fact that I opened myself up to "alternative" medicine (but how could I not after seeing the truth of the healthcare system with my own eyes.) I think it was my newfound realizations about living an intentional life that made me see the flaws in healthcare, or "symptom-management-bandaid-solutions"-care as I like to call it. Having this experience of gentle measures having great impacts opened me up to even more holistic thinking, maybe the mind and body really are one? Maybe everything we take in *does* matter, food, tv-shows, books, who we spend our time with etc. Maybe I heard about Ayurveda in perfect timing? The exact moment I was ready? I remember not exactly praying, as I was an atheist at the time, but thinking "I wish a healthcare system that saw you as a whole *human being* existed and which always did its best to heal the symptoms you felt, no matter what the blood tests said, and where you would meet doctors that *listened* to you without you having to fight to be listened to, and they had *time* for you." Soon after that I came across Ayurveda which checked all the boxes. It also eventually opened me up to the interconnectedness of all things, to God, the law of attraction, astrology, the kundalini and much more. My life suddenly became *magic*. I tried a kundalini meditation, because why not, I had a lot of time on my hands, and I saw a white light inside my head! According to yogic wisdom, Kundalini is a dormant life force waiting to be released at the bottom of our spines. Once awakened it travels up our spines until it reaches the "crown" (top of our head), and enlightenment ensues. I opened my eyes to check for the source, maybe there was a lamp in the room, but there was no bright light "outside" of my head! I closed my eyes again and my head began moving back and forth in a beautiful stretching-motion from the surge of energy I felt in my spine. I know, that must sound crazy but it happened. The world wasn't such a cruel, dark, hopeless place after all when I experienced that all of these things were *true*, I just hadn't been open to them.

I gradually opened up like a flower and reconnected myself to the beauty and magic of this loving, spectacular universe. I had been temporarily disconnected by the programming and trauma of our unconscious society. There are many things I do not understand, but I am so much more at peace, and I know that the help and information I need is always sent to me in perfect timing. I know that everything shitty is a lesson in some form that I am meant to master. I pass through shitty situations very quickly now as I immediately look for the lesson and in what way this is meant to upgrade me, be it in setting firmer boundaries, a chance to be brave or more authentic, a chance to heal past trauma, a chance to overcome an old fear, or a chance to trust the Universe more. We are not meant to stay stuck, we are meant to learn something and move on!

So after I felt better and more energized because of Ayurveda, I began noticing that the anxiety symptoms were still there and that the headaches and the loss of function in my arms and legs came and went in a *pattern*. Aaaaand the pattern was connected to when I was around my parents or other family members part of the toxic family system, or if I was doing or even just *thinking* about doing anything that they would disapprove of. My eyes would burn and my kidneys would explode in pain around my mother. I got panic attacks if I enjoyed myself, laughed or relaxed, or did anything I wasn't "allowed" to do. Keeping me in an extreme state of anxiety made me easier to control. I began realizing that *they* were the cause of my health issues and that they felt no guilt about making me feel this way or running me into the ground. I could easily have died TWICE and they would not have self-reflected on *why* Vera was dead or their part in it. They would not be seen as guilty or received any consequences from society. I would have been dead and no justice would have been served. Realizing this burnt through a lot of my brain fog and the false guilt I was carrying. I realized I would *die* if I stayed in contact with my parents and my family. *And* that what they had done was *outrageous* and *unforgivable*. They did not deserve a second more of my time.

It was around this time I came across the term *narcissistic abuse*. I surrendered to the rabbit hole and went on a ride through the internet and amazing books by Dr Susan Forward, Shannon Thomas and Danu Morrigan, and on the Reddit-forum r/raisedbynarcissists. According to the dictionary Merriam-Webster, narcissistic personality disorder is *"a personality disorder characterized especially by an exaggerated sense of self-importance, persistent need for admiration, lack of empathy for others, excessive pride in achievements, and snobbish, disdainful, or patronizing attitudes."*[1] I finally found descriptions of the manipulative patterns and mind games I had been subjected to for almost three decades. These patterns are apparently so common professionals have coined names for them. The guilt trips, the lose-lose-scenarios I was always put in, the shame I felt, how I felt so erased and how I felt way too much responsibility for my parents were all described in these books! Even the pattern that occured the most often was described perfectly in a YouTube video on narcissistic mothers I found by the coach Michelle Lee Nieves. She described a situation where a son was working on his computer, then the narcissistic mother would come in, ask him a question, then interrupt him and leave before he could answer. Why do they do this? Your upset is their heroin. These crazy behaviors are difficult to put into words, as the narcissist wants to hurt you without you being able to call them out on it. I will try to explain it with my own experience: my mother would seek me out and try to upset me on purpose, accusing me of something insane or make me feel dirty and sick if I told a joke. It could be the smallest things. If I told her about something funny I had told a friend in school, she convinced me I had told a sick joke and hurt my friend's feelings. If something broke, it was always my fault. If I made a small mistake, it was somehow catastrophic. If I threw a rock in the woods, we would probably find a dead child or a sheep around the corner and it would be my fault (this gem came from my father.) I jumped out from behind a dresser to prank my grandfather and she told me I "had been trying to kill him." She wouldn't stop until she pushed the right buttons. If the first accusation didn't work, she would change the subject three or four times, accusing me or criticizing me until she could tell I finally got upset. She would then get this satisfied smirk on her face that to this day makes me shiver to think about. It reminds me of Smeagol's grin when he cooks up an evil plan, from the Lord of the Rings. This happened forty to fifty times EVERY DAY and it was EXHAUSTING. No wonder I stayed in my room and tried to avoid her as much as possible! She was *feeding* off of me. My pain was her heroin and her satisfaction. I wish the therapists at BUP could have told me all of this when I was sixteen. Turns out it made perfect sense how these behaviors, done to me every day over so many years would wear me down and ruin my mental and physical health! I wasn't sensitive, weak, stupid or naive after all! I was a perfectly normal and healthy person trapped in an extremely toxic environment. All I needed was to leave, detox and become myself. I believe putting words to the confusing behaviors is a crucial step in recovery from abuse. Undigested trauma can then become digested, understood and archived instead of a gaping wound interrupting your day-to-day life. Also, researching narcissism helped me get out of the toxic guilt and gave me permission to cut these people out of my life. They were wild monkeys smashing up my windows and pooping all over my house, my house being my body and mental health, which means I am allowed to kick them out and set up stronger walls and windows so they can't come in. It's funny because as I was cutting contact and having all of the realizations, I had a lot of nightmares about break-ins, intruders and my stuff being smashed up, stolen or lost.

I also realized that I had been programmed to believe I was powerless and my parents, family members, teachers and the healthcare system had freely walked all over me. It was time to take my power back, trust myself and reclaim my life! In an ideal world people would hold themselves back from being shitty to others, but this is not the case, so *we* have to set boundaries and protect ourselves from unconscious and entitled assholes.

In May of 2019 I found an apartment to rent as quickly as I could. I had realized they were toxic to my health and that I needed to get out. I told my parents I needed a two-week break from them. This did not go over well as I was not allowed to have feelings and God forbid; *boundaries*. My father showed up at my door at my new apartment a few days into this break - which he was very aware of. He couldn't allow me to have any power to make such requests of him. Me displaying boundaries, autonomy and authority *outraged* him. He also couldn't let me have any *time to think*. When you have time to think, abusers lose control over you. He knew this. He was asserting his power and his territory. He was suddenly interested in me after twenty-six years of rejection, neglect and indifference. *They don't want you but they don't want you to be free.* He invited himself in and wrinkled his nose over my new apartment and left. I couldn't go two weeks without them coming to jab me with pain and shame. They also blew up other family member's phones trying to get information on me and my break from them. Their desperate tactics of control backfired as this helped me see their true colors even more clearly. I fluctuated between outrage over what they had done to me and certainty in the boundaries I needed to set. I was tortured by false guilt and believing I was selfish. And the thought of upsetting my parents felt life-threatening. In my panic I went to dinner at their house before the two weeks had finished. My mother insulted me around twenty-seven times in thirty minutes and I got the usual pounding headache as soon as I saw her hungry eyes looking at me.

I don't even know how she had the time to eat between her attacks! They triggered such anxiety in me that I couldn't sleep until 5 am that night. That's when I knew I had to cut all contact for life. Shakingly I sent them a letter which included a few short and clear sentences of how I knew I had been raised in psychological violence and that if they ever tried to contact me again I would call the police. I also returned their house-key in the same letter. I was so stressed out I passed out a couple times a day around this time. The support of a functioning mental health care system would have been great. I needed protection and guidance, but I had to figure it out on my own. I didn't reach out for any medical help because I was in such a fragile state that I couldn't risk them making the situation even worse. It didn't take many days before the *flying monkeys* swooped in. Flying monkeys are a term from *the Wizard of Oz* (book and movie) describing the henchmen that do the bidding of the Wicked Witch of the West. Flying monkeys are the enablers and the puppets of abusers, often abusers themselves. And now, ladies and gentlemen, here is the shitshow that ensued when I tried breaking out of the role as one of the family punching bags (there are more punching bags still trapped and I hope one day they also break out):

- My uncle called me and told me my parents were saying I was in a psychosis. And after faking concern about me he got me to tell him how I was feeling. And I was of course feeling *extreme* anxiety during attempting to break out of 27 years of abuse. He told me that what I was feeling "sounded like psychosis." But he didn't follow this up with any words of concern or something like "we'll get you help" or "I'll be here for you." Nope, he just wanted to hurt me. I don't think he would have cared if he pushed me over the brink to suicide. I will not lie, I was thinking about it. But I also felt like it would be such a *waste* to have been born into this life, be abused for 27 years and then *just die*. I wanted to live to see if life had more to offer. And BOY OH BOY, IT DOES!!! So please keep going!!! Anyways, I'm actually glad he said those things and revealed his true colors as a manipulator and abuser.

- My other uncle, who had shown absolutely no interest towards me my entire life, suddenly "wanted to talk." I declined of course! It's a little late to enforce your non-existent authority over me now... You had twenty-seven years to talk to me and build a relationship with me.

- My cousin's wife changed her profile picture to her doing a childish angry-face and tagged me in it. PLEASE don't marry people who perpetuate the same patterns as your parents. Don't marry emotionally immature people. You deserve better. I blocked her stupid face in real life and online. I considered if I should even mention her childish tactics in this book, as she doesn't deserve a response to her bullshit - but I decided to mention it so you can understand the overall load that was put on me. My family all attacked me simultaneously without any concern of whether this would lead to my suicide. I survived it and so can you.

- My grandmother pretended to faint after receiving a letter from me where I stated clearly the ways she had hurt me, and everyone accused me of trying to kill her. I thought she would be grateful for a chance to clear the air at her old age. And besides, being old isn't a get-out-of-jail-free-card for all the shit you've done throughout your life. She deserved to be put face to face with her negative ripple effects throughout the generations after her. The guilt trip didn't work on me this time though! They were *not* prepared for Vera having a spine! They all followed the behavior described in the books I read about narcissism down to a T and I could predict their every move.

It was of course stressful and horrible, but I felt like I had a secret guidebook throughout the storm. Seeing how they all banded together to protect the toxicity made it even clearer how my family is so sick it's *pathological*. I've found a lot of peace with this shitty grandmother after I confronted her (I have two abusive grandmothers, lucky me.) Even though she didn't own up to anything I feel at peace because I stood up for myself. I haven't spoken to her since, as the only way to have a relationship with her is if I pretend nothing ever happened, and that's not the kind of person I want to be. I have *real* and *healthy* relationships or *no* relationships. If she dies I will still be at peace. Because it was her decision not to heal our relationship. I did everything I could.

- My cousins invited me to a group chat with my mother and grandmother, giving them access to me after I had blocked them. I blocked all my cousins faster than you can say "enabler" after this clear display of disrespect and lack of empathy.

- Lots of other family members didn't say anything and did not reach out. Claiming neutrality in a situation concerning abuse is the same as siding with the abusers. It is unconscious, ignorant, hurtful and toxic. I blocked all of them too. There is such a thing as right and wrong. Morals are also a thing! We all decide what kind of people we want to be. I've decided I want to be a person who does the right thing even when it's hard. And I want to be able to go to sleep with myself at night and feel *peace*. To do that I can't have any wrongdoings of mine creeping in the back of my mind. But I guess we don't all have a conscience...

- One family member fully supported me and is cheering me on in my new life! Thank you!

It was a SHIT SHOW. And I survived it. And so can you. This temporary flare-up is standing between you and freedom. Run straight into it head first and burn down the dysfunctional circus! There was one more family member who told me "you weren't really sick, you made it all up for attention" and when I chose to begin sharing my story they called me "an attention-seeking child throwing a tantrum." And of course, accusing me of trying to "kill" my grandmother, as she is apparently too old to be held accountable for a lifetime of abusive and dysfunctional behavior. How convenient for her! To be able to abuse her children and grandchildren for decades and then claim to be "too old" to talk about it. Suck my dick is all I can say. I have chosen to leave the position of this family member out of this book as I still have hope for this person. I'm not holding my breath or waiting for them to heal. I am *open* but with appropriate boundaries in place until they prove themselves healthy and worthy enough of being in my company. I hope they one day repay me for my benefit of the doubt. I even called the police crying because I felt like I was killing my mom and that I was somehow a criminal. They were like "uuuummmm... Listen to me, you're 27 years old, you have every right to move out! Your mom is responsible for herself!" I needed to hear that I wasn't doing anything illegal from *the police*, and that's saying something about the level of brainwashing that had been done to me. It feels surreal that I survived all of this shit! And let me tell you, no one can frick with me after being gang bullied and abused by my family. I was shaky as hell, but I stood tall until the storm passed. They were SHOCKED that I wasn't easy to control anymore. I was terrified because I had been programmed to believe that they had so much more power than they actually did. I was terrified they would show up at my door, burn my house down, tamper with the brakes of my car, someone would commit suicide and it would somehow be my fault, someone would die because of "what I had done to them," get my apartment taken away, take the money out of my bank accounts etc etc. But it turned out, all they could do was throw adult tantrums and send me written bile. And *you can block phone calls, text messages and emails*. All they have are *words* and *you don't have to listen*. If they send you letters, throw them in the trash unopened or get someone you trust to read it first. Someone I trust opened my letters for me. I watched their face as they scanned the words. And I wish I could describe their facial expression as they read the letter from my "fainting" grandmother, it was HILARIOUS. This awesome person walked straight to the trash can with the letter, they didn't want me exposed to this poison! I picked it up because I wanted to read it to help me with my guilt and confusion. I kept it for a long time to look at every time I felt like the bad guy. It helped! Her insanity was written in black and white! This person's support helped me immensely. I hope you also have someone who can ground you in truth when you feel wobbly! We all need support and validation on our healing journeys. We all need confirmation from someone else that they see the same thing that we see. That's why I'm writing this book! To *validate*!

As I am writing about everything my family did, there is a part of me that feels scared and guilty. I feel the feelings and send myself love. There is no real threat. I was programmed to believe that truth is *bad* and if someone does something wrong and you call them out, then *you're* the mean one. But that's not how it works. They've had every opportunity to change their behavior, get help for their behavior, try to hold back their behavior, regret their behavior and apologize sincerely for their behavior. And I've seen none of it. If you walk around the city smashing windows you can't be mad when the police arrive and your face eventually ends up on the news. This is not my shame to carry. I hope this book helps bring this type of abuse into the light, so it can finally be transformed and eradicated. My wish is that my family and all others like it heal, and that society has knowledge about it, zero tolerance for it and the tools to help everyone involved instead of denying its existence and providing no actual help for the few people brave enough to ask for it.

aaaaaaaaaaaaaaaaaaaaaaaaaaaaaaaaaaaaaaaaaaaaaaaaaaaaaaaaa
That was a deep inhale. My story is long and sorrowful, I know, but it has a happy ending ;)

A few months after I left, I decided to try therapy *one more time* after talking to a friend who is a doctor. She gives me hope for the future of healthcare as she is very empathetic and intelligent. She advised me to write down my story on a piece of paper and just hand it to the doctor and wait for them to read it if it was too hard and overwhelming to explain the whole thing in five minutes. I met with my new doctor and handed her the paper. I nervously waited while she finished reading. "Wow, you've been through A LOT," she told me. It took me by surprise to be heard and believed on my first attempt! She immediately referred me to therapy. I was apprehensive, but since I was now best friends with the Universe and how "everything happens for a reason" I believed there was a possibility of a healing experience since I had now learned the lesson and had stood up for myself. There was no more need for the Universe to put horrible therapists in my path to give me opportunities to remember my power and stand up for myself. I was now aware of my power and my right to be treated with respect. I knew I was now capable of walking out mid-session if there were signs of there being a repetition of the previous bullshit. I was once again assigned a therapist, but for the first time my pain and experience was *acknowledged* and *believed*. I will never forget her. The funny thing is, she looked like an angel with her blonde hair, and to me she was. We had a few months together before she unfortunately switched jobs. We worked on exposure therapy together and she was very happy with the work

I had done on my own; voicing my pain in journals and letters, and confronting abusers. A family member even said "if you'd been to a *real* therapist before you sent that letter, they'd *never* tell you to send it," after I sent the letter to my grandmother which she supposedly fainted from. I wrote it from a recipe in a book by Dr Susan Forward called *Toxic Parents: Overcoming Their Hurtful Legacy and Reclaiming Your Life*. It was a great and constructive letter, voicing my pain and opening the conversation for healing and reconciliation! My family accused me of killing my grandmother while the therapist was all "great job, Vera!" when I showed it to her. LOL! Don't ever let toxic people advise you on what is right or wrong! They have *absolutely no idea*! And if I hadn't sent that letter, I would still be confused about my grandmother. She revealed her true colors and it allowed me to move forward with clarity and peace. Anyway, the beautiful blonde therapist taught me that fear shouldn't be avoided, but *faced*. Because *after* you have those new experiences there is *no more need for the fear*, it's gone! But you have to face *every* fear; confrontation only works on the specific things you're afraid of. This is "exposure therapy." We mainly focused on the fear of moving out and about in the city, as I was terrified of running into my parents or any flying monkeys. After a lot of repetition and hanging out in grocery stores with panic attacks this fear began to fade, and I came up with other areas I wanted to reclaim. I decided I wanted to wear a pink hair tie to reclaim my style and authentic expression. This triggered sooooo much shit in me. My mother's voice was tearing me a new one saying stuff like "you think you're pretty don't you?," "do you have some perverted obsession with the 80's or something," "you're trying to escape into an illusion instead of being a valuable member of society," "you're too old to wear a pink hair tie, wanting to means you have the mind of a child, you're sick" etc etc. I mean, all this over *a hair tie*. She used to tell me shit like this multiple times a day, so no wonder I had her voice on a broken record in my mind!

I put it on and went out about my day, just waiting for people to stare at me and roll their eyes. *And nothing happened.* NOTHING. HAPPENED. This was *crazy* to me! No one cared! I realized the only people who'll criticize stuff like this have *serious issues* and it has nothing to do with you. Normal people either don't care or they'll compliment you. So I gradually wore more and more of what I wanted to wear. A colleague of mine actually said "pink hair, huh… isn't that what four year old girls want?" after I colored my hair pink. I straight up left the room without saying anything, because I don't deal with such fuckery anymore. At that point I had healed so much that he couldn't rattle me. Just because he hates himself doesn't mean I have to! Each step was scary and each step was a *triumph.* Turns out, dressing up isn't *dirty* or *selfish*, it's fun and joyful! I apply this concept to everything I want to do now. I face my fears like the badass person I am!! Since then I've taken dance-hall dance classes (this is not ballroom dancing, it's a very sexy and cool form of dance originating from Jamaica with lots of twerking), I've worn sequin jumpsuits, colored my hair pink, put myself out there on Instagram and Youtube, moved to a new city and started school again at twenty-nine. It doesn't matter if I'm scared. If I want to do it I can, and I take the fear with me as we jump in together! I've befriended my fear. We're a team! And so my comfort zone has expanded greatly!

After the beautiful angelic therapist unfortunately switched jobs I was assigned a new one. The new therapist was really nice, but told me after a couple of months of shallow conversation that there was nothing more they could do for me since I was functioning so well. I mean, I was doing *okay*, but I didn't feel *deeply healed*. It felt like I once again hit a wall. Their main job is to *stabilize* people, they don't have the tools for *full* healing. Once again I was left to my own devices to figure it out. I knew I was not done healing, but I knew the Universe would provide me with all the necessary tools, triggers and situations to gradually continue upgrading and healing. And I knew I could continue with the journaling, feeling my feelings, and exposure therapy on my own.

I HEALED MYSELF

Let's rewind back to the summer of 2019, a few months after I had climbed out of bed and cut contact with my parents. When I was bed bound and listening to all the books on minimalism and intentional living, I came across Teal Swan on YouTube. Once again the internet provided me with answers. In one video ("How to heal the emotional body") she explained how you won't get trapped in your feelings forever if you stop running away from them. That's *how* you heal them. You have to *feel* them. And *let them finish*. The exact opposite of everything I had ever been told by my parents, health professionals and society. Once again I had that ding-ding-ding-moment of "this is what I've been looking for" just like with Konmari and Ayurveda. I am forever grateful to her for bringing me back to the truth I knew deep down, but had been searching for since the day I was born. Fireworks went off inside me! Finally! My gut was screaming *truth truth truth*! I began to see the value in spending some time feeling through the accumulated feelings I had racked up over the years.

I began trying to do this work while still living with my parents. There will be more on this in the "WHEN to feel your feelings"-chapter, but let's just say there was no point in healing old trauma while being filled up with *new* trauma simultaneously. But *after* I left, the floodgates opened by themselves in an epic release. Because my body *knew* it was finally over. I spent some time on my own, listening to emotional music and letting whatever that needed to come up come up. I flew to Italy by myself in June 2019, to *Eat, Pray, Love*-celebrate that I was out of bed and to conveniently leave the country at the same time that my parents would receive my break-up-letter. It was a beautiful trip that was hard to enjoy. I was freaking out and thought for sure I would meet my parents around every street corner in Sicily. But it was definitely the beginning of feeling my feelings. I locked myself in my Airbnb, put on some sad music and cried like I had never cried before. I cried because I had finally accepted the loss of the mother I should have had and which I would never get. I cried for myself. I cried for accepting that I was, and had always been, an orphan. I cried for what I had been through. I cried for what should have been.

After a couple of hours anger came up underneath the tears. I punched and pushed the air, defending myself for the first time in my life. I had never made these movements before. I would always freeze when I was attacked verbally or physically by other kids or adults. I had never *pushed* before. I couldn't scream or make noises yet, but I was beginning to push through all the sludge in my nervous system and push back in defense. It was physically hard to make the movements, like I was immersed in mud. My nervous system was so weighed down by trauma. It felt like I was punching and pushing the air in slow motion even though I was trying to fight like a boxer. But even though the punches felt weak, they were extremely strong. To find the courage to begin pushing back and standing tall after feeling like a skittish, unwanted disgrace hiding in the shadows who no one wanted around for 26,8 years, took courage lots of people will never have. Being abused by your own parents and having to fight them and cut contact with them goes against all our survival instincts and puts us in the line of fire of gossip- and the "this is how things should be and I feel entitled to tell you"- judgment squad. It breaks with society and is terrifying and unnatural.

But necessary. In reality, parents and grandparents, aunts and uncles abusing the children in their family is what is truly unnatural and does not belong in a civilized society. This gossip and judgment is upside down and targets the wrong people. I am gradually starting to feel like I'm not shunned by Norway as a whole and that there is still a place for me here. I do belong here and I am connected with the culture even though I was rejected by my family line. It was *only them* who rejected me. The rest of Norway doesn't really care, haha. No, seriously, most people don't care. In a good way! Most people know that some people come from abuse and therefore they don't have a family and that is natural. But it's more accepted if your parents were drug addicts, severely physically neglectful with food and hygiene etc., or physically/sexually abusive. Severe psychological abuse and emotional violence from "successful" parents is harder to believe. Your education, job, finances or status does not automatically make you a good person or a healthy parent. Norway (and the rest of the world) really needs to work on its "only parents without education abuse their children"-mindset. They do. And they hide behind this stupidity, naivety and denial. It's time for a psychological abuse cleanup throughout Norway and the world!

Since I now had realized that I had been abused, lots of repressed memories came flooding in. It felt like I had the task of digesting all the undigested emotions and horrible situations accumulated over twenty-seven years in front of me. Great... I embarked on the path of clearing out old emotions from my system and getting in touch with myself again. It was hard and I often wondered if it was even working as new pain up underneath everything I cleared out. The more pain I felt, the more pain came up. Was I running around in circles, creating more emotions? Would I eventually reach the bottom and feel good? I did. Your pain is like a heavy, filled-to-the-brim backpack you're gradually making lighter and lighter. I am still working through it, but I am now clearing out the corners and the hidden pockets of the backpack. I am finished with the main contents. I got through it with journaling and developing methods for staying with my feelings and not keeping myself constantly distracted, which resulted in this book! I really hope it helps you out! I hope it is already helping you out :) For all the suppressed memories that came up, I used the technique described in Teal Swan's book *The Completion Process: The Process of Putting Yourself Back Together*. It really helped me when overwhelming, horrible memories came up and I needed a way to "finish" the trauma and get some resolution without needing apologies from those who hurt me. Sometimes justice isn't possible and you have to find other ways of healing and moving forwards without suppression and unhealthy coping. Sometimes feeling the feelings was enough, sometimes the memory needed to be worked through, sometimes there was no memory, only feelings, and sometimes the same memory came up multiple times - healing different aspects of it every time. I will be sharing all of my discoveries in this book. Usually, the most powerful method when I felt emotions coming up was taking some time to myself, closing my eyes, letting the feeling intensify and waiting for a memory to come up. If it did, it usually was enough to just *look at it* again. I usually hadn't revisited the memory since it happened a very long time ago. Looking at it again made me realize I had drawn the wrong conclusions at the time, which led to tremendous release and relief. These conclusions were "they did this to me because I'm ugly," "my parents wish they had a different child than me," "there's something really wrong with me," "I'm stupid," "everything I say is stupid," "my social antennae must be broken," "I'm not athletic" etc etc. Revisiting the memory made me realize I was just surrounded by toxic people and that nothing no one ever did was because of *me*, but because of their own unresolved trauma. The kids in school, the dysfunctional teachers and unconscious therapists were projectile-vomiting their own trauma onto me. It wasn't because there was something wrong with my face or that I was somehow less valuable and less worthy of respect than others, it was because they *needed* and *chose* to do it to someone and I was *there*. I was simply just there. It could have been anyone else. It wasn't personal. I felt shameful about not fighting back at home or at school, but then I realized that I had tried as a little kid and since then I had always made the choices that would best ensure my *survival*. And I *did* survive. So I did an amazing job! It was very intelligent of me to put my safety first. I fought back at the perfect time when I was an adult and no one could feck me over legally or with any other form of control other than guilt trips and toxic letters (BURN THE LETTERS HAHAHA!) I forgive the kids in school as it was their parents' responsibility to not traumatize them and teach them healthy ways of regulating their emotions. I also made mistakes as a child. The adults who hurt me are a different story. They chose to be dicks to *children* instead of searching for ways to heal themselves; the ultimate laziness and lack of self-responsibility. I believe there comes a time when you go from child to adult and you have two choices:

go from victim to perpetrator

or

go from victim and onto a healing journey.

I know that *the how to heal* is not easy to find. But there are no excuses for *not searching* and *not trying* and instead traumatizing others multiple times a day for years. Abusers aren't even *trying* to do better. That's how you know it is a *choice*. I have been holding back from acting on pain and I've been searching for answers to find inner equilibrium since I was a very small child, so yes, I *do* judge people who aren't trying even though I've slipped up sometimes.

Even as a child I did better than all the adults I was surrounded by. They were not worthy of my old wise soul, my pure heart, my sunshine-energy or my jokes. Yes, I did flip my hair while writing this.

The third option you have when transitioning to adulthood (the first and second one being *go from victim to perpetrator* and *go from victim and onto a healing journey*) would be being stuck, holding back your pain and trying your best to not take it out on others, but not knowing how to heal. That's where I found myself for many years before I found out how to move forwards. It was a kind of limbo and a precursor to the healing journey because at least I was trying, but I didn't have the tools I needed to move forward yet. I was full of pain, trying my best to not be passive-aggressive or negative, but *damn* it was hard. I slipped up sometimes but I have apologized to those concerned. Sometimes I was a little toxic betch. It is never too late to own up to your behavior and apologize. If you feel guilty about something, try journaling through it before you take any kind of action. Find some clarity. And then apologize to those you hurt. It is very freeing. It's okay if they don't respond. At least you tried. There is a *huge* difference between *making a mistake* and *being a toxic person*. The difference is *taking self-responsibility or not*, and *trying* versus *not trying*. Sometimes we react, sometimes we're childish, but as long as you own up to it and try to do better then that's okay. Changed behavior is always the best apology.

Today my life is full of emotional intelligence. And it is SO SATISFYING. I am currently in film school and all we talk about is *emotions* and how to portray them, get the audience to feel them, and how to tell stories *clearly*. Emotional intelligence is a *necessity* in filmmaking. Every camera movement, camera angle, colors in the frame, costume, sound, or lack thereof, is chosen to invoke a specific emotion in the audience. The emotional rollercoaster throughout a film is carefully planned. My qualities are finally *valued*. I can use my emotional experience and intelligence, my ability to plan and follow through and my creativity *every day*. It feels so good after growing up in a home without truth, which instead was full of emotional pain and suppression. FREEEEEEEEEEEEEEEEEEEEEEEEEEEEEEEEEEEEEEEEEEE EDOM!!!!! I now trust the flow and natural progression of my healing journey. The Universe always brings in the right people, messages, tools and circumstances for my next step. Healing isn't a unicorn ride over the rainbow, but for every trigger and challenging situation there is a reward. There is pain and joy at every level. For every triggering person or situation, I know I am meant to master the situation and learn a lesson. Sometimes it is setting firmer boundaries, sometimes it is learning to let toxic people float by me and being unbothered (strangers, colleagues etc, NOT people you live with), sometimes it is taking action and leaving, sometimes it is standing up for myself, sometimes it is facing a fear and sometimes it might be learning patience with waiting for my dreams to come true. The lesson is NEVER to stay in toxic relationships or toxic situations, it is always about getting out of it and upgrading your life somehow. I believe that every time I state a wish or desire to the Universe, it will bring forth everything I need to heal to align with my desire. Which means there is always a small shitstorm before a breakthrough or an upgrade in my life. Sometimes *a lot* of emotions come up, I feel them, and then suddenly a few days later I am happier than I have ever been before or something I wished for comes true. I have learned to go with the flow and I remind myself on the "bad" days, aka the *healing* days, that they are only a precursor to the next amazing upgrade in my life. And it gets easier and easier with every step. In the beginning the triggers and emotions were like a thundering waterfall and I was standing at the bottom getting BLASTED (picture that, haha), now I deal with a small trickle. Healing takes a long time, but the intensity won't be as hard as in the beginning. At first you might need to do a lot of healing before you can function and live, and then it gradually transitions into more living and some healing work on the side. You can do this! Seriously, you can! One emotion, one trauma, one problem, and one step at a time!

To end off my story at this point in time, I'd like to reflect a little bit on the difference the therapists of BUP could have made to my life. How much pain, suffering and years lost they would have saved me if they knew how abuse works and had the inclination to ask me relevant questions that would have revealed what was going on, and had the guts to act on the information they would have found and the emotional and empathetic qualities necessary to believe me and validate me. Imagine if the *system* worked as it *should*. I often think about this. But now, as I am who I am and where I am, I don't know if I would have risked going back in time and changing any of it. I did lose ten more years of my life to abuse and had to go through hell in terms of chronic illness and pain, but I don't know if I would have developed the same level of self-trust and authority over my own life if I didn't have to fight my way out of it on my own. I don't blindly trust in doctors or any kind of authority anymore. I know the government and the healthcare system is full of damaged individuals who haven't worked on themselves or healed their pain before taking their current job, which makes me a healthy skeptic to everything they do. I am grateful for the clarity and the confidence I have gained. But I also know people can develop confidence from love and nurture too... And I also feel like my healing journey is just bringing me back to who I already was as I child, before the trauma and conditioning accumulated. I was a very funny, creative and energetic child before it got stomped out of me, and now it is gradually coming back. So was there any meaning behind all this suffering? Was it for a reason? I'm not sure! But I am where I am and it just keeps getting better and better so I'm gonna leave it there! Two and a half years after I cut contact with my family I have become a homeowner and a film student! I have *my own office* and I'm decorating it exactly how it looks like inside my head: vibrant colors, glitter and art! I'm in a happy, fulfilling relationship, I have the coolest, most supportive and kindest friends I could ask for. I am the most radiant and beautiful I have ever been and I don't think I've even reached my peak yet! As I am writing this I am planning a music video for a *real* debut artist. I mean, how did life even get this good?! The journey felt so slow, but then I suddenly ended up here! There was a looooooooong buildup before the breakthrough, so trust the process! Trust the process but don't be complacent. *Take action* on what your gut is screaming at you to do and say "screw you" to the rest! Thank you for reading my story! I hope it inspired you to trust yourself more and to take no shit! You can break out of *anything*!

CHAPTER 2

WHY You Should Feel Your Feelings

If you're here because you literally have no other choice, I feel you. Doing this work was my last resort and I *had to do it fast*. I was in so much pain physically, emotionally, spiritually, mentally, dentally, skin-wise, digestion-wise, ALL THE WAYS, that I needed relief *now*. My eyes even hurt. They were stiff, as if they had exercised too much. I mean what the FECK even is that. What a weird symptom! The pain was all-consuming and I couldn't do anything before I felt at least a little bit better. So let's just say I was extremely motivated. If this sounds like you and you just want to get to the good stuff, then please turn to page X for the "INSTANT RELIEF" section, where I have spelled out a simple process you can do instantly.

If you're not convinced feeling your feelings is a good idea after reading my story, then please let me do another pitch: do it for your physical health, your mental health and to be able to reach your highest potential in life. Let's start with physical health! Even though I know the orbital configuration of iron after studying chemistry for two and a half years, I am no scientist and I can't be bothered to find all the articles and reference them here, so you'll just have to take my word for it: science is now saying that repressed emotions aren't good for you. And stress. STRESS ISN'T GOOD FOR YOU. It makes you sick. Yeah, no shit, but thank you for researching this and please incorporate it into all healthcare systems, thank you! Past Vera would have been LIVID about me saying "science says" and not backing it up with a source, hahahahaha. Get with the times and feel your feelings! Let's start an emotional revolution! Let's end this dark age of shame and suppression!!

Let's look at an example of how inner work benefits chronic pain and the physical body. When I was twenty-two and still being abused, both my lower wisdom teeth got infected and had to be removed by surgery. The anesthesia didn't work at first and I had to get a double dosage. I still felt sharp pains during the surgery, but went through with it anyway because I didn't want to be rude or make a fuss... *face palm.* When the anesthesia wore off I experienced horrible pains and they lasted for weeks. I took strong painkillers and they somehow weren't enough. Fast forward to the fall of 2021 when I removed one of my upper wisdom teeth by extraction, one dose of anesthesia was more than enough! I didn't even feel the tooth coming out, the whole thing was over in no time and I didn't need a *single* painkiller in the hours or days that followed! *Not a single painkiller!* Not one! I know this wasn't a surgery like the other two, but I can also compare it to the innumerable (okay, maybe six) tooth-pullings from my childhood where I needed double doses of anesthesia and the painkillers never really worked for me afterwards. A deep connection with my body, feeling grounded, and deeper breathing was also waiting for me beneath the suppressed emotions. I also haven't had any more infections, not even a single urinary-tract-infection (which is very common for women, and at one point I had them once a month) after I started living more ayurvedically, stood up for myself and began healing my trauma in 2019. And since then I've only had the flu *once*. I've gone through some periods with less energy, but they all had explanations (going through grief, doing this emotional healing work and working a very hard shift-schedule.) I can't remember the last time I was sound sensitive. I don't feel cold all the time anymore. My breathing has improved immensely without doing breathing exercises. I also used to have a lot of sharp pains in my arms, and migraines. Both are almost gone. They only come back during *blasts from the past* aka when I feel triggered. So I feel like they don't really count and the intensity is constantly decreasing. And the best part: *energy*. My capacity in everyday life, and my energy, is at least one hundred times better than it used to be! It has increased proportionally to how much inner work I have done and also to what my nervous system can handle and deems *safe* after facing my hundreds of fears. I am slowly finding *flow* with my increasing capacity: I can do a lot, but that doesn't mean I have to! I know there is more to heal, but I have the tools! Wohoo!!!

If you have any kind of chronic condition, you're probably here because you've *already* tried everything to heal yourself. Or maybe you've been to therapy for years, read twenty self-help books, done all the affirmations and you still can't figure out why you're un-happy and in pain. I've been there. I went to therapy for three years which only left me with *more* confusion, shame and pain. I knew the therapists were missing something. And it is: healing. HEALING. IT'S HEALING. THEY DON'T KNOW HOW TO HEAL PEOPLE. And a lot of them don't care. They'd rather be right and hang on tight to their degrees and credentials than admit something is missing. Whew, that felt good to say! Like me, maybe you've experienced how incredibly shallow therapy can be. If it feels like a waste of time, maybe it's time to try something new! Or definitely switch therapists! There are good ones out there! You're allowed to be picky about your *health*! Maybe it's time to test out what happens if you run straight *into* your emotions instead of away from them. It's time to ditch the band-aid solutions and do some *deep* work so you never have to do it again! New emotions won't be stored in the same way as your old ones because you are now learning how to let them *flow* through you instead of accumulating them. If you do this work, you will benefit from it for the rest of your life. If you allow yourself to open the can of worms of all the suppressed emotions and traumatic memories - you will come out on the other side much lighter and able to live life from a space of true *flow* instead of *coping*. You won't have to *fight* through the days anymore, you will just *live*. Because you are in tune with yourself and can handle whatever is going on *right now*! Because your back is straight and your load is light. You don't have to handle the present *with* the heavy backpack full of past pain making everything harder than it has to be. It will be easier to try new things, you will have increased clarity and know yourself better, and it will be easier to take action on your dreams. Heck, it will be easier to find out what your dreams even are, because you've already begun going inwards and digging around! Life gradually blossoms! I thought inner peace and feeling whole were myths. They aren't.

Turns out, the only way to make feelings go away is to *feel them*. Shallowly talking about them, avoiding them with constant distractions, frantically exercising, overworking or tightening your stomach around them doesn't make them go away. Believe me, I've tried all of these and more. If we ever want to be able to relax and be with ourselves in silence, we have to feel through the pain. It *is* possible to be in silence with yourself and not feel pain, only openness, peace and joy. *And* to feel happy and joyful and have nothing pull you down or burst your bubble from the inside out. And it is all waiting for you on the other side of everything that has been repressed in your system. The lower you go, the higher you can go afterwards.

THE LOWER YOU GO, THE HIGHER YOU CAN GO AFTER-
WARDS

- Vera Wilhelmsen, lover of guinea pigs and self-quoter

Okay, now let's do one last pitch for the peeps in "the middle!" If you're not doing "that bad" you might think to yourself "why in the HELL should I put myself through feeling pain when I'm doing okay, I've moved on from that, I'm fine, I promise, I don't want to dig myself into a hole, why would I poke around in my past?" Well, let me tell you: if you don't go low you can't go high, be it on the dancefloor or in life. And feelings being a hole you get stuck in is a *myth*. A stupid myth drilled into your head during your childhood by toxic adults who lied to you so you wouldn't bother them with your "annoying" emotions. A brilliant method of control. If you don't feel the full depth of what you have stored you'll keep staying in this mediocre area of life until you work through those anchors weighing you down. Don't you want to know what your full potential looks like in this life? Don't you want to know how far you can go? How *high* you can go? How *happy* you can be? Don't you want to know what it feels like to feel *light*? To live with a light heart? To have *all* the options in life? To finally do the things you've always deep down wanted to try? Then please keep reading! Mediocre is safe, but it is also... mediocre!

YOUR FEELINGS AREN'T A PIT, THEY'RE A TUNNEL.

- Vera Wilhelmsen, sequin dresses-enthusiast, aspiring cat-mom and self-quoter

Emotional trauma is stuck in our bodies and is deciding our rules about life and what is possible for us. How? Have you ever had an instinct or a sudden impulse to sign up for a dance class or something *fun* or a little *"crazy"* (crazy according to the judgment-brigade), but then a new sensation washes over you and it is so painful that you think "okay, I guess not" and you end up not signing up, to protect yourself from more pain? *This* is emotional trauma making *very real* decisions for you *today*. Read that again!

EMOTIONAL TRAUMA IS MAKING VERY REAL DECISIONS
FOR YOU *TODAY*.

\- Vera Wilhelmsen, ice-cream connoisseur and self-quoter

If you work through it you will eventually only feel the urges and impulses trying to expand your life without any oppositional feelings pulling in a different direction. Traumatic and painful situations in your past get stored as energy in your body. When you want to do something that this past situation deems as *unsafe* because you previously got hurt, it will come up and scream at you to not do it. It doesn't want you to get hurt again! So when you acknowledge this, feel and breathe into it until it releases, then do it anyway. Repeat this process a few times and it won't come back anymore. If a memory comes up you might realize that situation wasn't your fault and doesn't mean you shouldn't do something or be a certain way. You were just in the unfortunate company of some toxic people, it had nothing to do with what you did or who you are. Something that was previously holding you back is now *gone*. The *energy* of that specific trauma disappears, and therefore the energy behind certain patterns is now gone. The patterns begin to collapse and gradually fade out of your life. The emotion has been processed, honored and released. You are now free to do new things, put yourself out there and *expand*. Imagine how fast you can evolve when you live like this? You'll be constantly upgrading every aspect of your life, constantly expanding your comfort zone, going after dreams that used to be only whispers, finding your unique purpose and voice in this world and actually using it. You'll be looking back and wonder how you got where you are *so fast*.

Right now you might be wondering "but Vera, I grew up with abusive parents and it wasn't just *one* situation, it was a megagigabeijingtokyonewyorkgazillion situations! Do I have to feel the feelings of a *gazillion* situations??? It will take me the rest of my LIFE!" No! I don't think it works that way. I grew up in abuse and experienced a bajillion traumatic situations until I cut contact one month before I turned twenty-seven. Now, two and a half years later, I feel good and light most of the time. The rest of the time I either feel fear from doing awesome stuff I want to do, expanding my comfort zone, feeling through leftover emotions, or simply feeling tired and overwhelmed from all the new things I'm doing. Not bad I'd say! In the beginning there was an almost *constant* purging of trauma and emotions. This lasted for maybe a year. I of course took "breaks" every day, and by that I mean it was impossible to fully rest with a nervous system in full mambo-jumbo-chaos, but distractions or focusing on other things did function as breaks, even though I didn't feel relaxed or happy. The pressure was *constantly* there to feel more, heal more. All my insides wanted was to purge and heal! There was so much that needed my attention and love to release! I had constant headaches from everything coming up which gradually lessened the more I released. I somehow semi-functioned as I had work and went to parties and stuff, but *all* my free time went into healing and feeling like shit. There were lots of moments of newfound joy in there as well, so don't freak out! It was a time of purging and new beginnings. Healing takes time overall and time and energy out of your day, but will also free up time and energy, and open up new possibilities for the REST OF YOUR LIFE.

In the beginning it didn't feel like it was working at all. But I didn't have a better method of healing at hand, so I kept going. After every release I immediately felt better, but it didn't last for many minutes before the next feeling came up. I usually took a break with some Netflix then. I didn't do multiple release rounds in a row, as I quickly found out this could lead to exhausting six hour sessions. That's not possible every day! I distracted myself to get a little bit of a break. Sometimes a release took me half an hour, sometimes it took me multiple days (more on this later.) It is important that you understand that it didn't take me two and a half years (where I am now) before I felt better - it took two and a half years to more often feel good than like shit! In the beginning I felt mostly bad and some intermittent moments of joy came and went to remind me to keep going - and gradually the balance shifted into feeling more good than bad. Now I go through occasional purges, and I don't have old feelings come up every day anymore! It's more like once every full moon and new moon! If I get triggered by something, I work through it. I don't have a definite answer on how long it takes to heal or if it is even possible to 100% heal, only that the more you do it the better you'll feel and the more your life will upgrade! Purge the old and simultaneously try new things such as new hobbies, going to new places and meeting new people. It's impossible to *not* make your life better if you do this.

IN THE BEGINNING I WAS IN ALMOST CONSTANT EMO-
TIONAL PAIN WITH A FEW MOMENTS OF JOY DISPERSED
INTO IT HERE AND THERE. THE BALANCE GRADUALLY
SHIFTED INTO FEELING MOSTLY GOOD WITH SOME HEAL-
ING OF OLD EMOTIONS HERE AND THERE. KEEP GOING.

- Vera Wilhelmsen, author of this book (which means I can do whatever I want such as use "LOL" and "hahaha" in a friggin BOOK!) and self-quoter, of course

Let's just say feelings and pain won't go anywhere until you go into them. So if you want to feel *better* you must first feel a little worse. And remember: you're not in a *hole* when you're emotional, you're in a *tunnel*, so keep going deeper and you'll find the light again at the bottom! It will all be worth it when you come up for air, and can take a deeper breath than you ever have before! *Nothing* is permanent or written in stone. Absolutely nothing. I used to believe I had a certain type of psyche and certain moods. I thought I would be depressed and suicidal for the rest of my life! I used to believe I had chronic, incurable illness. It was all bullshit from professionals who didn't know how to dig deep! I have transformed my own psyche from the inside out, without force, "pulling myself together" or suppressing my feelings, which transformed my life externally, and I want the same for you. Here's a hug! Hope you can feel it. See you in the next chapter! x

CHAPTER 3

WHEN You Should Feel Your Feelings

So, by now I've probably convinced you to cleanse your body and soul from the sludge of your past, but I also want to leave you with some insights on *when* it is beneficial to do this work. Sometimes it might be wise to focus on other things *first* or to first put some conditions in place.

If you're living in abuse, make a plan to get out and *then* start processing afterwards. Put your focus on the practical side of leaving and starting over somewhere else *first*. How are your finances? What are some baby steps you could take towards financial independence? Are you eligible for support? Can you save some money? Or sell something? And are you *safe?* Is it safe to leave without dangerous repercussions? Can you make a plan with law enforcement and healthy people you trust? I tried to begin the healing work while I was still living with my parents. I did experience amazing emotional releases - but- and this is a big butt (see what I did there?)- for everything I released through the front door, I was filled up through the back door with *new* trauma. Wow, this really turned into a butt-metaphor... There's no point in trying to heal the wounds while you're still being stabbed. Stop the stabbing first. I also hoped I could heal and still be in contact with them. But it doesn't work that way. It was only in long amounts of time *without* them and their stress I could really see them clearly. It was while not being in contact with them I experienced *peace* and realized just how much unnecessary drama and stress they were creating. They chose to stress out and abuse others (their children) as an insane coping mechanism, no matter the consequences to others instead of healing. Me staying and enabling them definitely wouldn't help them evolve nor heal. If so, all the love I had already poured into them would have done the trick. Not to even begin describing the detriment to *me* and *my* life! You can't sacrifice yourself for someone else when it is *their own* responsibility to help themselves! Don't let people stab you. Period. Periodt. With an extra T! It takes up way too much of your time and energy to process all the unnecessary drama and emotions, and to spend your time thinking about what they have done and trying to predict their future reactions is such a waste. Life is too short for this. Did you know you are allowed to *only* be in good relationships? *Crazy* right? Imagine what you could do with all that extra time, energy and mental clarity? You could make *every dream you've ever had come true* instead of being stuck with these abusive broken records. Try *blocking* the stabbing instead by not being in contact so you don't have to constantly heal. Don't take poison again and again and the antidote again and again – just stop taking the poison!

DON'T TAKE POISON AGAIN AND AGAIN AND THE ANTIDOTE AGAIN AND AGAIN – JUST STOP TAKING THE POISON!

- Vera Wilhelmsen, self-quoter because this is so damn important I wrote it down AGAIN

If you're *not* in contact with any abusers, toxic people or energy vampires, or only experience this very rarely or on the periphery (such as at the grocery store), then always feel your feelings. If you can't do it on the spot, like at work, then try to take ten minutes in the bathroom to breathe through it or journal, and/or feel through it when you get home. If the feelings need more time than a bathroom break, then acknowledge them and let them know that you would feel them if you could, and promise to get back to them later. If you forget, that's totally okay! They will be triggered again sooner or later naturally. You will get to them eventually!

The best place to feel your feelings is in the safety of your own home (with no toxic people) and the best time is when you are either home alone or when you have at least an hour to yourself. And since this work requires quite a lot of energy, don't do it right before a big event or anything similar. You might need a nap afterwards or a chill evening or morning at home before you rejoin the world. I usually do it before bed or in the morning. I go to bed extra early so I have time to journal or to feel if anything comes up! In the morning I do a much shorter process, such as ten minutes of journaling and then feeling through the feelings as I move around and get started with my day. More on this in the waking up in emotional pain section.

So let's feel our feelings and let's not create new buildup! But don't obsess about this or think that feeling your feelings is some kind of extreme math equation you always have to make sure is balanced. The Universe will always make sure stored emotions are triggered and healed at a later time, so don't worry about making sure you build up NO stored emotions. Go with the flow! Nothing is meant to be *that* hard!

CHAPTER 4

INSTANT RELIEF - Try This First

So, here are my two main methods for healing:

First, lay down on a bed or a couch. It's better to lay down than to sit as it opens up your chest and stomach more than sitting does, which allows your emotions to move more freely. Next, try to go limp. And by limp I don't mean you have to fully relax, but just open up a little bit in the stomach and chest area to see what comes up. Let whatever comes up roam free and keep your awareness on it as much as you can. A tightness might emerge when you do this, which is fine, as that tightness *is* something coming up for healing. Let it intensify and follow it around with your awareness. Simultaneously, let your breath do whatever it wants. You might feel an urge to hold your breath, breathe very fast and hard (similar to "breath of fire" from Yoga) or take really deep breaths. This will change as you go. The main point is to not control the breath, but to follow it wherever it wants to go. Think of it as allowing your nervous system to restart and cleanse itself, it needs to be left alone for a little while while it does its thing. If you feel an urge to retch or burp, allow it. Old energy is being purged from your system. YOU ARE DIGESTING AND RELEASING POWERFUL ENERGY FROM AN EXTREMELY TRAUMATIC EVENT STORED IN THE BODY UNTIL NOW. TRUST THE BODY AND ALLOW IT TO FLOW THROUGH YOU. KEEP GOING YOU BRAVE BEAUTIFUL PERSON! If you feel like rocking back and forth, do it. If you get a headache or any kind of pain or physical symptom, let that intensify too. You'll never get to the bottom of it if you don't dive deep into it. It intensifying while you're feeling emotions is a sign that it is connected to repressed emotions and trauma. I used to get lots of headaches when I felt triggered or felt any kind of emotion. I had to stay present with emotions and headaches to learn they weren't dangerous, and the more trauma I processed the less headaches I had. The whole point is to step out of the way and let your nervous system reset itself. Whatever you feel or think, meet it with compassion and have a conversation with it. Imagine it is your inner child coming to you with this pain or problem. What would the emotion or tightness say if it was your inner child? Healer Candace van Dell always says you should give your emotion a voice! Maybe it would say "I'm scared," "I don't want to be here" or maybe "oh my god, oh my god, everyone will make fun of me and hate me if I do this!!!" Make the subconscious conscious. Try to get the emotion to talk and keep it talking until it feels satisfied with having expressed itself! Maybe it needs some words of encouragement and validation from you. If no words come, that's okay too, it's just *one* method of many. Stay in bed and feel until you feel lighter or feel like you've completed something, or for at least thirty minutes. After you feel a little better, take some deep breaths, fill up the tissues that were holding emotion for years with fresh oxygen. If memories or images come up in your mind, let them. Watch the memory play out and feel the feelings connected to it. Journal through it or use the method described in Teal Swan's book *The Completion Process: The Process of Putting Yourself Back Together* if you need more work on it to feel closure. After the memory has played out is usually when I have some sort of aha-moment about a belief I've been carrying since that specific traumatic situation happened. Such as "everything I say is stupid." This belief disappeared after working through specific memories! At the time of the trauma I usually came to the conclusion that it was my fault and that there was something wrong with me. Going through the memory again as an adult releases that shame. Processing trauma unlocks wisdom, confidence and relief.

The second method that has immensely contributed to my healing is *journaling*. And by journaling I don't mean writing down what I did today, I mean dumping whatever I'm thinking and feeling down on paper until I feel better. The paper should need therapy after you're done with it! I've found that journaling can be very helpful in discharging emotions when it is simply too hard to be present with them, or in addition to feeling them in the body. The method is to simply write whatever comes to mind until you feel relief. It does not have to be written neatly, make sense or be read again. You can throw away the paper afterwards or keep it. Destroying it afterwards will help you write more uncenscored! I have saved a lot of journals as they remind me of how far I have walked on the path back to myself - but since I switched to ripping up the paper once I'm done I have been able to get more down and dirty into the things I'm ashamed about or afraid of looking at. You can also voice-record instead of write! Find what works for *you*! You can even doodle patterns with your pen that feel like they express the emotion you are feeling. You can doodle an entire page black if it feels good! Whenever I feel overwhelmed, anxious, indecisive, sad or angry I journal! If you feel stuck you can try beginning with describing where you feel tension or an emotion in your body. Keep writing whatever comes up after that. Validate your pain, speak to yourself as you would if a small child experienced what you went through. A couple of questions that might help you go deeper: what was I just thinking and is that 100% true, who made me believe this? And ask yourself "why?" until you find the bottom or core trauma, and journal and feel through it!

Here's a journaling example from my life that might help you: I used to have a lot of trouble with falling asleep before my boyfriend was also in bed. I even felt angry and resentful if he wanted to stay up later, without knowing why I felt this way. I could not relax until everyone else was asleep. This is what I journaled:

I feel so anxious at night. I don't know why. I feel completely fine, even sleepy, and then it suddenly goes away when I go to bed. It's so annoying! I AM tired, but then it passes as soon as I get into bed and is replaced with this weird anxiety. I feel angry when he doesn't go to bed at the same time as me, this makes me feel like a crazy person! Why can't I fall asleep before everyone is settled down for the night? (At this point I closed my eyes and waited to see if something came up.)

Memory: I am in bed. It is very dark. I feel small. I think I might be seven years old. Everything feels so big and the world is coming down on me, swallowing me, crushing me. I am listening for footsteps. I need to be awake so I am prepared. My mom can come running into my room at any moment, to "check" if I have fallen asleep, but in an aggressive way, or to accuse me of something I've done wrong or not doing something I should have done, which I didn't know about. It's better to stay awake so I don't have to come out of sleep before I have a defense or apology ready to tell her. If I take too long it will be too late and she will use it against me. If I take too long I will drown. She will say something and it will be so painful that it will take hours before I can feel my body again. I cannot take another sleepless night. I need to function in school tomorrow. My dad can come running down the stairs at any moment. I feel so scared when he runs towards me. I know he does it to scare me. To shut me up. To control me. Just the sound of his footsteps terrifies me. They don't care if they make noises and wake me up, so it's better to stay awake until they're asleep than be woken up, spin out (I didn't know what panic attacks were at the time, and it felt like spinning out), *then wait to fall asleep again. It takes such a long time to fall asleep after they've woken me up. All the sounds they make scare me. What's wrong with me? Why can't I just fall asleep? Why am I so sensitive? I am a bad daughter for being scared of my parents. How mean of me. They never rest. They are always coming for me. I need to be awake because the wolves are awake and they are on the prowl.*

No wonder I couldn't sleep until my boyfriend was in bed! I was never fully safe enough to sleep until my parents were asleep! They really were on the prowl for the kick they got out of scaring me and keeping me on edge. They *knew* some angry footsteps would terrify me. I had already done a lot of healing work when this memory came up, so I didn't write down any validation, as I easily give it to myself internally while the memory is "playing," but if I were to have journaled through it it would have looked something like this:

I am so incredibly sorry that you had to go through this, Vera. It wasn't your fault you were afraid. Your reactions were completely appropriate to the situation and your previous experiences with your parents. They were unsafe and unpredictable. They did not act like parents. They scared and mistreated you on purpose and took pleasure in your reactions. Your nervous system did a perfect job of keeping you alert and minimized pain and punishment. It WAS better to prepare for an attack from your mother rather than having her catch you off guard. You knew you couldn't leave so you protected yourself instead.

You survived in the best way possible! I am so sorry you had to be on guard, and especially to protect yourself from your own parents. I am so sorry you couldn't get quality sleep or enough sleep. You were a child and you needed and were entitled to sleep. It was their responsibility to make sure you got enough sleep and that you felt safe, happy and loved every day and night. They failed spectacularly. You never have to sleep at their house ever again. You will never sleep in an unsafe environment ever again. I will protect you and make sure you are only surrounded with quality people. I am so proud of you and I am so sorry.

I haven't had trouble falling asleep alone since this memory came up! I don't feel abandoned if my boyfriend wants to stay up later anymore. And I feel less anxious if I am woken up by a noise and have to fall back asleep. This process can also be done inside your mind, but it might be wise to do it on paper until you get the hang of it! Happy journaling!

You can do both journaling and feeling when the emotions need more than one method. In my experience, I've found that journaling first and then feeling through the rest, or feeling first and journaling through the rest both work. So experiment and find out what works best for you!

Let's summarize!
Feeling through it:

1. Lay down.
2. Go as limp as you can and let whatever comes forward come.
3. Let your breath do whatever it wants.
4. If you feel like doing any kind of movement, let yourself! You are expelling old energy!

5. Stay there until you feel relief or the emotion coming out of your throat. Try to stay with yourself for at least thirty minutes.

Journaling

1. Write whatever is on your mind or describe how you feel.
2. Write or doodle until you feel relief.

Some questions to help you work through it (ask yourself inside your mind or write it out in a journal)

1. Ask "Why?" until you get to the bottom of it, and journal and feel through what you find there
2. Ask yourself "what was I just thinking and is that 100% true?"

If memories come up:

1. Allow them. Rewatch them without interfering until you feel like you have seen it all.
2. Feel through whatever comes up. Allow all the feelings, also anger and rage!
3. Be open to realizations about what happened such as "wow, that wasn't my fault after all!" This will help you release shame.
4. Validate and comfort the you that went through this. Talk through it in a journal or in your mind.

Other tips:

1. "Give the emotion a voice" - Candace van Dell on her YouTube channel. Keep it talking until you feel relief. If it

wants to be quiet that is okay too. Tune in to the needs of your inner child.

2. See the "Here Are The Tricks!!!"- chapter for more ways to trick yourself into feeling your feelings ;)

That's it! This is mainly what I do and what I have done to heal myself, plus the book *The Completion Process*, and facing my fears, which we will explore in the "Triggers" chapter!

CHAPTER 5

How to Know When You've Succeeded in Feeling Your Feelings

There are four ways in which you can measure your success on this journey:

The first one is *relief*. Sometimes when reaching the end of feeling through an emotion, I would feel it coming up and out of my throat. I would often cough, burp, retch or feel an urge to do some deep exhales. After that I would sometimes feel an urge to laugh, feel an almost orgasmic feeling in my entire nervous system and sometimes a short moment of silence before the next emotion hit. Sometimes I felt lightness and relief, and sometimes I felt nothing and wondered if I had just wasted three hours. But I hadn't!

The second improvement you might notice is being able to do things that previously were triggering, without feeling triggered. Things that used to be super hard are now easy and simply feel normal for you. Or being *less* triggered even though you still feel triggered. An example for me would be when it suddenly became normal for me to go to dance classes and leave it all on the floor, whereas before I would have never gone in the first place out of fear of upsetting my mother. This took many dance classes and the improvement I felt was very gradual. Dressing myself in the morning without anxiety was also a huge improvement!

The third measure of success is suddenly being able to, and being interested in trying new things. This is an *amazing* sign! It means you have some extra energy and that your life is slowly expanding.

The fourth way you might notice improvements is through symptoms or ailments becoming less intense or even disappearing! Is your appetite better? Are you less constipated? Is your digestion better? Is your skin doing better? Your hair? What about those head-aches? Did they disappear without you noticing? Are you sleeping better? Are some areas in your body less tight or tense? Do you rely less on medicine and painkillers? Is your hair growing out thicker? Do your nails break less often?

I did not feel all of these simultaneously! It was a long process with lots of ebbs and flows! Sometimes I didn't feel like I was seeing any improvements, but I kept going and then they suddenly came a month or two later! You're not going too slow! You're doing great!

CHAPTER 6

Don't Force It!

Something I've learned in life is that thing's aren't supposed to be *that* hard. Simple usually does it. Health isn't *that* complicated and it doesn't require complicated, expensive solutions. I mean, I wasn't sick because I was *lacking* insane amounts of vitamin B or tea from a rare mushroom from the forest (yes, I did spend a lot of money on "chaga" mushrooms.) Reducing stress, becoming yourself, processing trauma, moving your body and eating stuff from the fruit- and vegetable section from the grocery store usually does it. Nothing wrong with super-foods or health products, but don't rely on them to heal you or force them down in large amounts. They are more of a bonus and a health boost rather than a necessity. My point is, if something gives you a feeling of drowning in complicated regimes, maybe look for something else. If you have to keep on taking in something then it isn't a cure. If you're stressing out trying to heal with a daily program of twelve different breathing exercises, yoga, foam rolling, epsom salt baths and hypnosis or whatever you do, read this word and tell me how it makes you feel: *simplify*. Does it feel like an exhale? Simplifying while working at the *root* (trauma and emotion) might just be the thing that gives you the energy or health you're looking for. All the planning, checklists and routines I had were *exhausting*. Have some fun. Have some orgasms instead. Dance. Play. There's nothing wrong with a challenge that helps you grow, or the tough beginning phase of learning something new (I had to put in effort to learn Ayurveda, I read books and made changes to my diet, I figured out what my symptoms were trying to tell me), but drop the things that feel straight up impossible or like suppression, blockage or going backwards. Such as shallow advice like "let go of the past," "forgiveness is a gift you give yourself" and "this is Peter, he recovered from chronic fatigue by doing ice baths every morning at 4:30 am." If something feels impossible to keep up with in the long run, then either adjust it until it becomes manageable and possible to integrate into your flow, or drop it.

After I left abuse and moved into my own apartment, I wanted to get into a healthy exercise routine *really fast*. But stretching and exercise triggered so much fear in me. I would tense up and become sore the next day without even getting started on a workout. I just couldn't do it. It wasn't the right time for me. I could go to dance classes even though I felt triggered, as I had to focus so much on the steps that I forgot about my fears. But as the 'rona hit and dance classes were put on hold I tried to run and work out at home. I could rarely follow through with it. Now, two years later, I can go for runs without getting triggered. I still don't have an amazing exercise routine, but I walk a lot every day and do yoga, strength and dance classes on YouTube at home here and there. I feel like this area of my life is *slowly blooming*. It's okay to take your time. It's okay to let things evolve. I needed more healing in my nervous system before I could exercise and stretch. I needed to feel, process and journal first. I needed to feel safer. I needed to figure out some stuff first. If something feels too hard, then wait and do other things in the meantime. Work on what you can work on *right now*. Sometimes when you do work in one area, it benefits other areas without you even trying. Feeling my feelings improved my digestion and appetite, facing my fears during the day helped with my insomnia at night, going to dance classes helped me un-traumatize my sexuality etc. Cooking, cleaning, exercising and creating a routine felt *impossible* for a long time. I continued feeling my feelings, journaling and facing my fears and they gradually began falling into place on their own.

Mindfulness meditation triggered horrible headaches and panic attacks in me. For a long time all I could do was journal, feel feelings (it *is* meditation, but in a different form, which didn't trigger me in the same way), and sometimes I did some chanting or went to group meditations. I definitely felt like I wasn't doing enough, but it was *more than enough*! It moved me forwards at the perfect speed! By chanting I mean yogic mantras, such as the one I mention later in this book, in the "Additional Exercises" chapter. It brought up a lot of emotions in me, so I paced myself. I did it both alone and at *kirtans*, which are group singing meditations/worship in Bhakti Yoga, which is a branch of Yoga. Meditation is not a one-size-fits-all in what someone needs overall or what someone needs on a given day. Sometimes all we need is to be still and feel through whatever needs us, sometimes we need to do some *work* on it to break through such as what's described in Teal Swan's book *The Completion Process: The Process of Putting Yourself Back Together*. Sometimes we need *parts work* (or "internal family systems work"), and sometimes when meditation is too hard, journaling can be the medium which helps you work through the tension. Sometimes we need silence, sometimes we need release and sometimes we need to communicate with our inner world so it can express release and find new perspectives. Sometimes we need to punch a pillow or scream in our car on the highway. And sometimes we need a new external experience to learn that something is safe or doesn't work like we were taught. Such as me experiencing how no one cared if I dressed like I wanted to.

Only doing mindfulness meditation didn't get me anywhere as it didn't let me work *through* anything. Focusing on breathing when emotions and traumatic memories were screaming was extremely triggering. Now, after a lot of inner work I do it for focus and stillness, but when I was full of pain that needed me, it only felt like suppression and self-abandonment. Changing your focus from the breath or from trying to find stillness, to your *emotions* might help a lot! Notice how the feelings intensify, shift and move around. The feelings will be there until you honor them. They need to be fully felt and move through your system to go away! You can meditate all you want, but unless you address your emotions and your trauma you will never find the happiness you seek. It's waiting for you on the other side of processing your past, so you don't have to carry it with you anymore! You can start doing mindfulness meditations when you have processed more trauma, it might work better for you at a later time!

When you are walking the path of the inner healing work, I want you to know there are no rules. You don't have to find the perfect balance. If you feel like you need to spend six hours in bed crying, then do so! If you want to dive deep and feel for hours until you feel better, then do so! If you don't feel like doing it today, then don't! If you feel burnt out from the inner work then take a break. If you've been in bed for an hour feeling your feelings and you still don't feel better, and you're beginning to stress out over the things you'd rather do, then go do them! Every minute you feel and release counts and adds up! Don't be so hard on yourself. You're really trying to heal! I think *flow* is a better word than *balance*. Balance implies you have to find a perfect middle path. But that's impossible! Flowing between both sides works too! Simplifying and removing pressure is alfa omega!

The planets are always moving into new positions, triggering you, bringing up emotions to be healed, and helping you have the aha-moments you need to move forwards. Certain breakthroughs, such as with cooking and cleaning will be easier during certain planetary positions. I love following astrology accounts on Instagram, it always helps to know I'm not going crazy, there's just a retrograde of some sort, haha! If something is just too hard right now, wait for a better time. Pay attention to what feelings and patterns are coming to a head right now, and try to heal those. You have to work very hard on staying stuck for a long time, because the Universe *will* force you forwards, be it with conflicts reaching a climax, putting you in situations where you *have to* make a choice, closing doors you shouldn't walk through or opening better doors. I believe becoming sick and having to break up with my family and quit the forced career path I was on, was a part of my Saturn return. Saturn will break up everything that isn't authentic and isn't supposed to be in your life. It will increase the pressure and make your life a shitstorm so you can step up and become who you are meant to be. Find ways to remove yourself from toxic and negative environments, step into your power as captain of your own ship and your own healing journey and the Universe will help you by putting you in the right situations for the next step and putting the right people, messages and tools in front of you.

If you're worried about *everything* you have to heal, the countless kilograms of traumas and insecurities you have in your backpack, "how will I even get through everything? How do I even discover everything I need to heal?" Don't worry! You don't have to dig, or map out everything you think you might be carrying. Just work on what you're struggling with right now, and the next thing in line will come up by itself soon! It's the same thing with patterns: figure out the pattern you can see clearly right now, try to put it into words and work through it, and wait until you see the next one clearly and then heal that too. Just learn the tools and use them on whatever you're currently feeling, you don't have to look for things to heal. FLOW BABY.

About Hard Times...

What about hard times such as break-ups, divorce, grief, loss and breaking up with your family? Should we attempt to process them and move on from them as fast as possible? In my experience, feeling the feelings, journaling and processing as much as I could helped a lot, *but* they took a long time anyway. But it probably would have taken a lot longer if I didn't take the time to do the inner work. It's been two and a half years since I broke up with my family and I'm feeling pretty good, so I definitely healed most of my trauma in quite a short amount of time! So yes, we should try to process them at a speed that feels genuine while also accepting that it will take some time. I don't believe we always need to be in the perfect balance, so if you're in a lot of pain and you want to feel better *fast*, then do as much inner work as you can until you feel like you need a break - then take a break, and repeat. Ebbs and flows.

Some feelings can be felt through in an hour but some feelings need to linger over us for weeks and months. For me it worked to do processing and healing work for two hours almost every day. I was in so much pain that I needed to do it to feel better as soon as possible as it was very hard to function, so this might be too much or too little for you, depending on your situation. With some feelings I felt instant relief, but I also went through periods of overarching sad fogs that could last for up to three or four months. These feelings that don't pass easily will pass after they have lingered for a certain amount of time. You can find more about these in the "Here Are the Tricks!!!"-chapter. I went through multiple of these grief periods, at least I think they were about grief. Flow is an important word here as well. They came and went on their own. No matter how hard I tried to make them go away, they just did their own thing. Feeling and journaling helped me a lot, but at times there was nothing I could do except hang in there until I eventually felt better. Sometimes it felt like journaling and feeling wasn't working at all. But, it *does* make sense that I felt really sad, down and like life was meaningless after fighting to survive in abuse for twenty seven years and then standing pretty naked in life without a family and realizing that I didn't get a childhood. It was heartbreaking. I felt broken, damaged and dirty. But I allowed myself to feel it and that's probably why I feel better now. I *moved through it* and I still am moving through it, but it's a lot easier now. The worst is over. And now I harvest the fruits of my hard work in a new city while I pursue my dream career!

Allow the feelings, feel them, distract yourself when you need a break from the healing, take care of yourself and do healing work as much as you can, while also not forcing your way through it and trying to make it pass as quickly as possible. It needs to suck for a little while. The more you let yourself be in a hard time, the quicker it will pass. The more you distract yourself the longer it will take.

Obviously eat, sleep, have a life, don't just feel and wait till it passes if you feel like you want to be out and about. And if you don't feel like going out and having shallow conversations while you are doing this life-changing inner work, then don't! Listen to your gut and do what you need to do! But don't do it to distract yourself from pain. You're allowed to grieve, you're allowed to go through a shitty time after a breakup or a loss, be it a person, job, home, situation, whatever it is, you're allowed to feel it and be in it. It's okay to gain or lose weight, it's okay to not be on top of groceries, cooking, cleaning etc. for a while. Take care of your pets and your kids, but other than that then watching six Disney movies and eating a pack of cookies for dinner might be good for you hahah. It's the fastest way through. If you allow yourself to go low you'll naturally want to start climbing back up because then you've felt it and now you feel ready for something new. After a couple of days of not leaving my apartment and having survived on porridge and cookies, I naturally wanted to take a shower and tidy up a little. I didn't want to watch any more Disney movies as I had already done that for three days straight. I wanted to shower and go outside. I climbed out of it without even trying! Let things flow! Every time I have "let myself go" I have naturally risen afterwards. It's time to release the toxic fear we have been programmed with. We do not need to tightly control ourselves. We don't have to stand over ourselves and criticize and whip ourselves like our old school teachers did, because no one is inherently lazy. You aren't! You don't have to tightly control yourself to make sure you don't fall into an abyss of junk food and depression. Try to let go of the control and see what happens! I found out I had natural urges to clean, shower, eat more vegetables and go outside if I didn't do so for a few days. We *do* have instincts. When the pendulum swings a little bit too far in one direction, we'll naturally want to balance it out. If I eat too many sweets one day, I can't even stand the thought of them the next day and will crave something healthier. These instincts became stronger within me the more I listened for them and the more emotional baggage I worked through. If you feel like you don't have any limits to your junk food eating or similar right now, that's okay. It will come. Work on connecting with yourself through the practices described in this book and give yourself time. It's always most efficient in the long run to work on the root cause, aka emotions and trauma, rather than doing band aid solutions such as affirmations (without any emotional work), "going outside" (it can't fix everything, lol), yo-yo-dieting or extreme exercise regimes that can't be upheld in the long run. Allow yourself to fall apart and you will naturally piece yourself back together and get back up again, feeling better than before!

Triggers

Let's talk about being *triggered*. I have no idea what the scientific, medical official definition is, and I don't care, but I see triggers as an unhealed wound from the past being poked in relevant situations to that wound. Under every trigger is either a feeling that needs to be felt, a memory that needs to be worked through, a fear that needs to be faced, or all three. I used to get extremely triggered by criticism, even when relevant, constructive and delivered nicely, as my parents used to constantly and unfairly criticize me. I had a *huge*, painful, aching wound around criticism. I am still working through this, but it is now a twinge instead of a gaping wound. I also used to get triggered by Miley Cyrus, which is so funny since I am now a huge fan of her. Her freedom triggered the pain I felt around not being free. Now that I'm free she doesn't trigger me and I love watching her do her thing, it gives me energy instead of triggering pain! (This is why I can share my story so openly on the internet, because I know that any negative comment that comes my way is about the commenter's own wounds, and *not* about me.) Being around people in general was also extremely triggering for me, be it going to the grocery store, being at work or being around friends. I had experienced so much trauma in close relationships and people felt *unsafe*. I will describe two methods for healing triggers here, and they are both equally important and must be used *together*!

Triggers *can* be worked through and they *can* be healed. A combination of processing and getting new experiences have worked very well for me. So in the case of being afraid and anxious around people, working through my trauma with feeling and journaling (as described in the "Instant Relief"-chapter) *and* going out there and being around people even though I didn't feel like doing so and it was horrible while doing it - healed me. The more I did it the safer I felt! I needed *new experiences* to rewrite the story of "everyone's unsafe" to "some people are unsafe and I can easily avoid them and set boundaries against them." I learned how to face my fears and get *new external experiences* from the angelic therapist I mentioned in my story. Don't avoid triggers, *face* them instead! Fear won't kill you. Sometimes I felt so triggered I worried I was going to collapse or become so tired and shaky I would be frozen to the spot and somehow get stuck in a grocery store and the employees would have to mop me up from the floor. But to this day it has *never* happened and I used to have *serious* complex PTSD. Even if I did feel myself going over the edge and getting triggered into oblivion, I stayed in the situation and within thirty minutes I could use my legs again!

Fears have to be *faced*. They cannot all be overcome sitting on your meditation pillow or in your journal. Because you won't know if the world works in a different way than your fears, or if your fears should be listened to or not until you go out there and *experience* the world. What happened to you was a very limited part of the world, done to you by very specific people. Most people are nice, warm and treat others with respect. We can recognize and heed red flags, use our old experiences as protection when necessary, and also let in the love.

So, when we're triggered we:

1. Feel through it and/or journal as described in the "Instant Relief" chapter, and we...
2. go out into the world and face our fears like the brave little ducks we are until we get so many new experiences that we finally feel safe!

In my experience, some triggers required the first method and that was enough, while with other triggers journaling and feeling didn't work at all, only getting new experiences worked, and some triggers were healed by a combination. Experiment on yourself! This experimentation also leads to getting to know yourself better which is great! Yaaaaas!

Try the two methods mentioned first, and here are some other tips for when you feel triggered into outer space:

- Move. Just shifting a little in your seat might be enough. This helps to remind you you are *not* powerless or trapped, you *can move around*. Like "oh, that's right! I have a body with muscles which means I can get the feck out of here if necessary!" This often leads to remembering I can leave, say something or take some form of action, do something new. Take a new path instead of what I usually do. It takes me out of freeze mode! Remembering I have the power to leave, say something and take action makes me feel safer. It helps me shift out of autopilot and gives me the option of trying something new and getting a new experience.
- Sit your butt down, take out a journal or do a voice memo. Say whatever comes to mind, recount what happened when you felt this way before, describe how you feel, say whatever you want to say to the peers in middle school, your parents,

the teachers, the school system, the parents of your class-mates, your ex, say it all. Don't hold back! When you feel done talking or writing, or if your hand cramps up, but you still feel emotional, lie down on the floor and fully surrender to the emotion, let yourself fully "die in it." Stretch and shake. If it's really hard, I find that a combination of being still and shaking works, alternating.

- Write out what you think is happening and how you feel. Get in touch with that traumatized, maybe younger part of you that needs to express itself. It thinks the same thing is happening right now *in this moment* as what happened before, so meet it with love and help your inner child take a look around and realize you're in a different place, in a different time, and you're also an adult with free will who can protect it.

- This is really hard, and I'm not perfect at it, but when I feel triggered by people I try to ask myself "did they really say it how I heard it?" before I react. Sometimes it was just an old wound that came up and they didn't really say anything wrong. If it's in my inner circle I ask them like this; "this might just be trauma, but can I just ask you if you meant X in Y way? I just need to know." Sometimes I wait and gather more experiences and data with that person until I decide if they are toxic or not. And sometimes the red flags are so obvious I take them seriously straight away and begin avoiding said person. But since I can sometimes be sensitive with healthy people, I wait and see until I feel certain about them and their inten-tions. You'll figure it out for yourself with enough experience (I tried to insert a heart emoji here, but apparently you can't do that in a book...)

- As mentioned in the "WHEN You Should Feel Your Feel-ings,"- chapter; if you are out and about when you get trig-gered or overwhelmed with emotion, take a couple of minutes to yourself in the bathroom. Close your eyes and let the emotion intensify. Let it do whatever it wants until you feel it coming up and out with your breath. Shake it out! You might also become an expert on feeling your feelings after some practice, and you can walk around feeling your emotions in public with a poker face, no one will know! :)

Good luck! x

CHAPTER 9

HERE ARE THE TRICKS!!!

I promised you tricks, and here they are! And here is a tiny refresher on *why* we are suffering through this: remember, *you are not in a hole, you are in a tunnel! Feel your feelings, dig deeper, feel MORE until you come out on the other side, into the sunlight.* The more you feel, the more you journal, the more you process - the better you'll feel emotionally and mentally, the more clarity you'll have and the more grounded in your body you'll feel! The more you journal the more you will get to know yourself, and because you know yourself you will be able to create an external world that feels better to your inner world.

This chapter contains the tricks I've discovered on feeling the feelings that don't pass, and I have sorted them into the following categories:

Stretches

Massages

Miscellaneous but Important Tips

Breathing

Writing & Inner Work

What Was I Just Thinking?

Is This a Current Feeling and Not a Repressed Emotion?

Taking Action

Let It Be

STRETCHES

Some emotions are very difficult to breathe through and release, they feel like stuck tar, aren't responsive to breathing and don't "move." For the most painful and stuck emotions, such as numbness in your lower belly, that drag on for hours and you feel like you're not getting anywhere; yoga poses can help get them moving and eventually release. The stretching creates a pathway up and out your throat and helps the breath penetrate them better.

Please look up these yoga poses online and try them out. Hold them for as long as you can or for as long as it takes to get the emotion moving.

EXTENDED PUPPY POSE

FROG POSE

RECLINED BUTTERFLY

THE WHEEL: can't be held for long as it requires a lot of strength, but it might get you started. It will bring attention to tight areas in your stomach and chest. Transition to one of the other poses if you begin with this. It takes a lot of strength and it is not necessary to hold this pose for long. If you notice strained or shaky breathing in this pose it is an indicator of emotions that need to be released, especially grief or hopelessness/despair. You can notice your progress in this pose, as there will be less and less tight areas as the months pass on your healing journey.

COBRA POSE: This is a powerful hip opener. Widen your legs until you find the emotional sweet spot, aka when you feel *worse*.

THE BANANA: I made this one up. Put a pillow or multiple pillows under your back, lean back so you turn into a banana, opening your stomach, chest and throat.

For all of the stretches: let yourself cramp up, convulse and shake, don't force yourself to keep the posture. Lay down, curl up in a ball or begin moving around when you feel like it. The whole point of this is to get you back into your body and tapped into your intuition - and process the past of course. The convulsions help move the emotion up and out. If your emotion just lasts and lasts and feels stuck then get in one of these yoga poses on your bed or on your mat and see what can happen in thirty minutes! This has worked wonders for my most painful and stuck emotions. The deepest feelings of hopelessness were trapped in my lower belly, blocking me from deep breathing throughout the day. Meditation and trying to feel and release them wasn't working and dragged on for hours. This area felt dead and numb. Stretching out the belly in some sort of mild backbend seems to do the trick in my experience. Curling up like a ball might make the feelings milden and get sort of hidden but stretching out really does the job for the *release*. You can curl up in a ball to invoke a feeling of safety. But if you feel like it is blocking the emotions, then open up in a backbend. Put some pillows under your back and relax backwards in a curve. You can alternate between curling up and bending backwards on your bed.

In my experience, backbending too far might block the convulsions and shaking that comes with some emotions, so I would recommend only the mild and medium belly stretches and backbend poses. This is quite exhausting but deeply healing work. Do this on a day where you can rest and nurture yourself afterwards. If you do it before work or an appointment because you simply have to, then tell yourself you are proud of yourself and do something nice, nurturing and relaxing for yourself later in the day. Sometimes we are in such emotional pain and we have to move through it before we start our day, maybe after a nightmare, so do it! You might feel exhausted right now, but doing this work will free up more energy in the long run. Nightmares often play out scenarios that bring up repressed emotions that need to be released. I always do my inner and emotional work in the morning because I'm forced to, but this might be different for you, start trusting yourself and build a routine around what makes *you* flow.

You might also feel intense waves of energy or numbness or heaviness moving through your legs or other areas of your body. Let them and don't stop. Weird sensations, such as heavy energy, can also be repressed like emotions. If you stop then the emotion was only halfway processed and you'll have to pick up where you left off later. That is of course okay, but for your own sake please try to keep going! These sensations won't kill you, they have been stuck in your body waiting to be seen and trickle their way through your nervous system and eventually dissipate.

MASSAGES

- Massage your solar plexus or any point of tension that feels numb, dead, tight or like the epicenter of the emotion. Rub the spot that feels the tightest to help the emotion loosen and move. Pound it until it begins to open up if necessary. Keep rubbing as it moves to a different place. It might go through a series of locations in your belly and chest before it eventually releases into the lungs and you can breathe it or sigh it out. Typical epicenters of emotions are in my experience anywhere along the large intestine, the sacral chakra (an energy center under your belly button), the solar plexus chakra (located over the belly button) or heart chakra (in the middle of the chest.)
- Take a shower. Let the flood of water hit the tight spot, or your stomach or chest if you don't know exactly where the emotion is stuck. The warmth might help the muscles relax and the emotion to begin to move. The heat and the steam might also help you begin to breathe, which also kickstarts the process. Stay in the shower for as long as you feel like if you have the time.

- You can also try EFT, "Emotional Freedom Technique," or "tapping" on harder to reach, deep emotions. There are tons of videos you can follow along on YouTube. EFT did not work very well for me, as I ended up tapping until I got tendonitis without feeling any better. It also triggered a lot of panic in me, as I tried it in my very early stages of trauma recovery. But I do believe different techniques work well at different times. I sometimes just tap on my chest and it makes me cough up some tension, which is nice! It can really get emotions moving! Tapping on a specific point instead of following a routine around my body worked better for me. It is definitely a technique worth checking out! If it makes you tense up and feel more afraid, and doing it for fifteen minutes doesn't make it better, and now you're just frozen in tension - then it wasn't the right technique for you at this moment. Try tapping at the center of your chest instead. I used to feel way too triggered to remember the full technique. Simple usually does it. Tap where you feel pain and tension to help the feeling move. You'll feel it when you hit the right spot - what you're feeling will intensify. When using massage or rubbing to move an emotion, do not tap or rub until you get tendonitis! Switch to a different technique before you feel pain! I sometimes go through many different methods while I process an emotion. And remember, some emotions can't be processed in one day. But you are always moving through layers. There is always progress. After I finally said goodbye to my family I had to grieve the loss of what I never had and what I never would have and also grieve the time taken from me lost to abuse and not being allowed to live my own life. I had to grieve the loss of career, loss of identity, loss of freedom, loss of happiness and relaxation and the pain of living in such survival mode for so many years. Let's just say my sadness, anger, grief and numbness couldn't be worked through in fifteen minutes. But all the minutes I spent processing over many months added up and I feel so whole and happy now! :)

MISCELLANEOUS BUT IMPORTANT TIPS

- Making sound helps:
  Say aaaaaaaaaaaaaaaaaaaaaaaaaaaaaaaaaaaaaaaaaaaaaaaaaaa and change the frequency until it hits the spot and reverberates through your emotional tight spots. Change the frequency (go higher or lower) until you feel like you are singing out your feelings.
- Scream and swear in your car on the highway. Or in the forest. Or into your pillow.
- If some feelings feel especially difficult to move through your system then get up and start shaking. YOU ARE YOUR OWN SHAMAN AND YOU ARE GOING TO HEAL YOURSELF. Shaking is such a relief. It's like shaking the nervous system clean of old tensions and old energy. You start out feeling in pain and stuck and end up feeling light and full of feel-good chemicals. Turn off the lights and shake and crawl around in a dark room if you feel self-conscious. Move however you want and for as long as you want. You can alternate shaking/dancing and lying down on the floor to fully surrender to the emotion. Start shaking again when you feel a little better.
- Start dancing. Try expressing how you feel through dance. Change your movements until you feel them enhancing and expressing how you feel. It's not supposed to look good or

smart. It's for your nervous system, not for the opinion-firing-squad. Search for ecstatic dance tracks on YouTube if you want to be accompanied by music. Search for ecstatic dance events in your area if you want to take it a step further.

- This one is gonna sound a little weird, but you're already in uncharted waters here, so why not, you might be surprised if you try it. Lay down and *put a crystal* on your third eye, on your forehead between your eyebrows. Or on your chest, or any of the chakra points along your spine. Feelings will intensify. I don't know anything about crystals, I just buy them using my gut feeling and also choose which one to use during my healing-feeling-sessions with my gut feeling. After I put it on my third eye a feeling usually intensifies, I breathe into it for a while until I feel where in my body it is the most intense, usually somewhere in my stomach. I then move the crystal there and breathe into it until the feeling releases. I then move the crystal to another tight area and breathe through that area. I do this until I feel like there are no more tight areas or I *have* to do something else, like use the bathroom, eat or get on with my day. Remember, *everything* you release *counts*, even if you didn't have more time for healing today, you still made your emotional backpack lighter and your body healthier! Good job!

- Do energy healing on yourself: push up energy from the depths of your stomach, and up along your esophagus until it comes out of your mouth by breathing quickly or clenching and releasing your stomach rapidly. Let yourself retch and burp (don't do this right after eating.) When nothing more comes up then take some deep breaths in to reoxygenate.

- Have someone hug you. It might make the stuck feeling move upward so that the tears can come. Or hug yourself, hold yourself, *be there for yourself* like those who let you down should have. We are frozen in fear and painful emotions just like when we were children because *no one came*. No one came to help us process our emotions. All these years you've been waiting *for you*. And here you are loving yourself, healing yourself. You are doing an amazing job! Here's what I do: I hug myself, really *hold* myself for how long it takes. I *contain*, or *envelop* myself until I feel better. And I let that inner voice express itself if it wants to. I *hug* and I *listen*. It is very important to stay there like you have no other commitments or stuff on your to do list. A child won't open up to you if they can sense you don't really want to listen to them. You have to hold yourself and let yourself feel the emotion for as long as it takes. If it takes hours it means you're not making yourself feel safe enough to process. When we feel safe, the emotions move quite quickly, in minutes or in half an hour. Signal or say to yourself that you will be there for as long as it takes, that you aren't rushing, you aren't abandoning or have more important or better things to do. This can look like holding yourself tightly with no intention to let go, having no *time limit* on the hug. Kissing yourself, rubbing your arms like you would rub the back of a child processing emotions. Tell yourself *you* are here now and you have the power to give yourself *everything* that wasn't given to you. Everything you should've gotten. Tell yourself "everything can be rescheduled, everything can be moved to another time. *You* are what's most important."

MUSIC

- Imagine yourself in a music video or a movie. This is just a part of your story, the hard part the main character of a movie goes through. The hard times will eventually become good times! This phase is character development! Romanticize sitting with your pain to trick yourself into spending some time on it. Put on some music that enhances how you feel and stare out the window on the train or the bus. Have a main character-moment while driving. Recognize the *magic* of it. You are literally CHANGING YOUR LIFE RIGHT NOW. YOU REALLY ARE.

- Put on the saddest or most angry music you can find. Listen to something that *enhances* how you feel. Happy music is great, but it won't cheer you up, that is *suppression*. Listen to the happy stuff *after* you have felt through what you were feeling, because you *will* feel happier afterwards. You do not have to force anything. Here are some songs that help me feel my feelings:

- For anger and empowerment: Bullet for My Valentine - *Waking the Demon*. Bullet for my Valentine is a band that in my opinion has a lot of songs with amazing lyrics on psychological abuse. I'm a huge fan and have been since I was a teenager! This song is especially powerful, as in the music video there's a victim of bullying who stands up for himself. It also reminds us that anger is empowering and not something "bad." Try listening and punching the air or a pillow. Feel your strength and power coming back to you, stand up to your bullies and those who took advantage of you. They made a *huge* mistake. They messed with the wrong person.

- For grief: Desiree's *I'm kissing you* helps me cry (it's from the 1996 film *Romeo and Juliet* with Leonardo DiCaprio.) This always gets me crying.

- Listening to music from a difficult time in your life might also help to bring the emotions up from stuckness to fluid tears. What music did you listen to when you were a child, teenager og whenever you went through a hard time? The other day I spent a couple of hours listening to music I liked during my teenage years, it brought up a lot of grief which I sighed out multiple times over two hours. I sat there until I felt lighter. I had moved through it. I don't feel the same heaviness when I think about my teenage years anymore. I've also listened to music I listened to during my 20's, and I felt a lot of love and heaviness for the young woman who was so trapped. But this young, but a little bit older woman, is now free ;)

BREATHING

- If it doesn't trigger you into oblivion: take deep or short "pumping" breaths while laying down, sitting, walking or moving until you have released the emotion. This works for me *now* after years of inner work and coming back into my body. Like I mentioned in the **"Don't force"** section, I journaled and faced fears first. Breathwork might be very triggering after trauma as the forcing of the breath might feel like a boundary violation. I sometimes start with breathwork and then transition into however I feel like breathing to release on my own. You can do a couple of minutes of breathwork and then transition into a different technique of emotional release, *there are no rules*. There is no rule that says "thirty minutes of breathwork or no breathwork." Remember you have full autonomy over yourself now. You can stop practices at any moment. You are not trapped or ruled over. *Flow* instead of rules.

- Look up "breath of fire" online. It is a yogic breathing technique.

WRITING & INNER WORK

- Write letters to the people that hurt you. Or the people you have hurt. Send or don't send them - completely up to you. But write it as if you are *not* going to send it, as this will make it easier to be more honest. I used to feel the need to have a confrontational conversation with my parents, but after writing it out in multiple letters in my journal the need disappeared. Writing it out before taking action can help you get clear on what you want and need. There are no right and wrong answers here. I see a lot of advice in the narcissistic abuse recovery community about not confronting the abuser because it will drain you. As you might remember from the "my story" chapter, I did send a letter to my grandmother which was not well received, but it gave me peace anyway. If it is safe to confront, then do so if you want. It's okay to be drained after doing something big. Just don't go back over and over again to "talk it out" because you hope they will change. You can totally say everything you've ever wanted to say to them, drop the mic and then block them afterwards. Up to you! And if you make a mistake - so what? Then you gained some experience which you will benefit from going forward!

- **Speaking to your inner child** in a nurturing and loving way may be very helpful. As a child it is likely that the feelings *did* go on forever and ever because you were always getting a fresh fill of abuse and neglect day after day, year after year. Did you feel like time passed very slowly in your childhood and like you couldn't wait to grow up? I certainly did! Remind your inner child that you aren't in that environment anymore, and that you have/or will set boundaries that will ensure their safety going forwards, and that feeling these feelings will actually help this time. It was pointless to process these feelings in childhood as we had no control over our environment or what happened to us. I remember lying in bed at night as a child feeling horrified and in so much pain, feeling that pain was never helpful as it only kept me awake and would weaken me for the next day where I would need to be hypervigilant. I couldn't waste precious energy on being anxious or crying about something that had happened when I knew a hundred bad things were coming tomorrow as well! Reminding my inner child that this is not the case anymore really helps. You can also try stroking your own forehead or chest while you feel these feelings. This is the nurture that you should've received as a child which would've really helped you regulate your nervous system. We need touch and love, it is an integral part of relationships. It is never too late to give this nurture to yourself and slowly open yourself up to receiving it from and giving it to others.

- Say to yourself: "it's just trying to move through my system." This might make your muscles relax more and provide more free flow through your system and a quicker release.

- If **memories** come up then play through them in your mind and see it from your perspective now instead of what it was at the time. You might realize you weren't to blame after all and it wasn't your fault. Or maybe it was a shameful memory and now you realize you didn't have anything to be ashamed about! Feel the emotion fully, go through what happened if a memory surfaces and feel the relief of your new conclusions. If you gain clarity on something *you* did wrong, which can also surface, then first make sure you aren't taking on responsibility that isn't yours by journaling or talking through it with a friend. Sometimes there is no conscious memory. If so, let the feeling pass through your system. Focus on it, go deeper into it, let it intensify and move around.

- Sometimes clusters of memories will come up and you might feel very strong emotions for hours or the entire day. If the process starts happening while you're at work or similar, then say to your inner child "I see it too! I promise I will fully deal with this when I get home, I won't forget, I promise!" Feel as much as you can, but also go on with your day and try to go for a walk or get some movement in when you feel like it's too much. Let yourself mourn and process as much as you can.

- Look into "parts work." Another name for this kind of work is "internal family systems." This work lets you access suppressed parts of you and have a healing conversation with them, removing resistance, blockages and tension. Teal Swan has a great, free YouTube video on this which explains and demonstrates how to do this by yourself. Search for "parts work" online. Sometimes you need a *conversation* with your inner parts, to *solve something*. This also ties in with Candace

Van Dell's amazing quote "give the feeling a voice!" Talk through stuff - with yourself!

WHAT WAS I JUST THINKING?

• Ask yourself what you were just thinking. I'm willing to bet 99% of our thoughts are broken records saying things that aren't even true. Thoughts we aren't aware of are trains running uninterrupted in our minds. They usually pass unnoticed in the background and suddenly you feel like shit. "I'm all alone," "my life sucks," "I have no friends" etc. Is that 100% true? Most thoughts aren't even true and we need to interrupt them with our awareness so that thought-track gradually gets used less and less and eventually dies. Talk it out or write it out with yourself! Give it a voice and have a conversation with it!

TAKING ACTION

• Is this feeling a *current feeling*? Some feelings aren't from the past, they are *current*. What does it want to tell you? Some feelings need to be taken action upon. Maybe your inner child is sad that you never have fun anymore? Maybe you're feeling lonely and should call someone or schedule some quality time? Maybe you're in a toxic relationship or in a job that isn't aligned. Being in the wrong place or career creates constant feelings of sadness, fear and depression. Maybe you're feeling the vibration of your neighborhood, building or city? Some places have a cap on how happy it is possible to be within them in my experience. The matrix is just *so heavy* in some places. It takes experience to be able to read your feelings this well. Give yourself time to fine-tune your inner world and to find out what feelings are from trauma and what feelings need to be taken action upon. If you don't have clarity then wait before you take action.

- Maybe you're tired or overwhelmed? Simplify your schedule or take some days off until you feel better. Can you eliminate something that's draining you?

- Are there any **external** aspects of your life you need to take control over in order to feel safe and happy? Finances, grocery shopping, cooking or showering? Can you improve some of your basic needs so you can trust yourself to take care of yourself? Self-trust can be *built*. Are you feeling frozen and not able to take action in your finances? I've been there. Try taking some small baby steps even if they trigger you. Baby steps really do add up! Log into your bank and take stock! Can you make a simple plan going forwards? Build one habit at a time.

LET IT BE

- *Get on with your* day, allow the feeling to be there, let it over-arch whatever you do. By doing this you are still honoring yourself and your feelings, even though you aren't sitting still with them. Process it with your breath as you go about your day. And once again, you don't have to take perfectly deep breaths! Maybe the emotion will come out in a sigh. There are no rules. Let it stay there with you as you do your thing, maybe that's all it needs. Imagine the feeling as a baby koala on its mother's back, just hanging out. You are the koala mama and the emotion is hanging out on your back, following you around, feeling loved and important being allowed to come along with you! You don't have to do anything special, just allow it to be there! Know that some feelings will stay for days or weeks. They just need to be heard and know they are respected, and you do that by allowing them to be there. They need to be honored for a specific amount of time which only they know. Tap in and out of them as you go. Your best is more than enough.

- Wait and see if you just need to experience this situation a certain amount of times until you realize it is now safe and not threatening.

- Sometimes I was sad for WEEKS. And it felt like nothing was working. I journaled, I felt, I went for walks. I did *everything*, but I still felt sad. And then it suddenly passed! On its own! It just had to hang out in the part of my nervous system I was conscious of for a while - where the pain was. I didn't need to dig for memories or to analyze it! It needed to be heard and honored. It didn't need anything else than just some *time*. Grief takes time. It isn't only death that leads to grief. Allow yourself to feel grief even if you feel you "have no good reason to." Your feelings don't care about your stupid rules. They still need to be felt ;)

- Check the calendar to see if there's a new moon or full moon coming up in a few days. This might sound *w0oWo0* but a lot more emotions will come up to be released during the days around the new moon and the full moon. Embrace these times of the month as healing days. Excellent days to do inner work, as you'll be forced to anyway. Might as well go with the flow!

- Sometimes it isn't the right time for a certain emotion or a tense spot in your body to release or come forward. If you can't get through, then wait. It will come out for healing when certain conditions are in place or when it's ready. Don't force it! Go about your life, heal what you are currently aware of and everything will fall into place!

CHAPTER 10

Pass-Out-Level-Fear aka Being Triggered into Oblivion

Now, I'd like to talk to you some more about getting so triggered you feel like you might pass out or get stuck somewhere. When you feel so triggered that you feel like your fear has shot you beyond oblivion and far into outer space. My mother loved to keep me in this state of extreme anxiety, as she would get her fix both from seeing me suffer *and* the opportunity to tell me how stupid I was for being afraid. I would get so tired from being so scared all the time that I used to fear getting stuck in shops and malls. She would then talk about my fear in front of strangers and family friends. Lovely. She put me in this state and then made fun of me for being in it. Fear and panic will come like a wave. If you let it increase it will eventually peak and begin to go down again, like a rollercoaster. But you have to be brave and let it increase. If you try to avoid it or make it go away, you only extend the stage it is currently in. It will pass in the shortest possible amount of time if you let it fully do whatever it wants. Focusing on my hands and feet while I let panic flow through me usually worked for me. The more I did it, the smaller the amplitude of the curve became and the shorter the duration became. If you know a little physics or have ever seen a diagram of a sound wave, the amplitude is the height of the wave. The amplitude gets smaller and smaller the more you feel your feelings. If I fully let fear flow through me then the whole thing is usually over within thirty seconds. That's how practiced I am at feeling feelings now! It's pretty great and very practical!

I'm not gonna lie, I *have* passed out from fear a couple of times. It happened during the first two weeks after I cut contact with my family, where I imagined all kinds of horrible repercussions. I feared for my life and for the "legal power" they had made me believe they had over me, even though I was twenty six, soon to be twenty seven, almost a decade older than eighteen, which is the age you become a legal adult in Norway. But it only happened when I laid down on a sofa or a bed. I was so terrified that I dissociated so hard that I woke up a few hours later. I know I didn't sleep as adrenaline was pumping through me, I went somewhere else. I have no idea what happened. I think I passed out or somehow went out of my body. I felt the same level of fear when I was out walking, grocery shopping or whatever I was doing trying to get through this horrible time - but I *never* passed out while I was outside or doing something. And I never got stuck in a store or a mall, no matter how scared and tired I was. I think I "went away" only when it was safe to do so. We are geared for survival, and passing out when it isn't safe isn't beneficial to survival. But use your own judgement of course! Maybe build up gradually with driving and heavy machinery on your healing journey.

This fear was extreme and I should definitely have had the support of a therapist or doctor during this time, but they do not have the tools or understanding needed to help abuse survivors. I also had no idea how to explain to them what I was going through, and I knew they wouldn't be able to help me find the words. I was also afraid anything I told them could be used against me, as it had in child therapy. I was afraid they would deem me "crazy" and side with my parents. It's heartbreaking how I went through this alone. But I survived. And it got better. And I hope this book serves as a companion for others going through the same thing or *anything* alone.

The only thing that really helped when things were this extreme was to hang in there and see how everything played out. It took weeks and months, but I experienced that the only repercussions came in toxic messages, letters and phone calls from flying monkeys, which I could block. They had no legal power over me. I checked my car for anything suspicious, such as the brakes being tampered with, for *a long time.* I bought my first car after cutting contact with them and I seriously believed I would be rejected in garages and repair shops, that the people who worked there would tell me things like "you're not allowed to have a car because you are an incapable little girl" and then take it from me, I kid you not! But once again I faced my fears and did all the car-things even though I at first felt like a stupid little girl who had no business doing such things. Eventually this feeling passed, I learned more about cars and my confidence grew. They couldn't take away my apartment or the money in my bank account. I began to see my family for what they were, immature and abusive children instead of monsters with all-encompassing power. Their power was an illusion they wanted me to believe. It was brainwashing. My fear gradually subsided because time passed and they couldn't do anything to regain control over me. I didn't lose a single friend even though my family spread horrible rumors about me. They couldn't get me fired or influence anyone other than their own toxic circle to not take me seriously or to not respect me. I realized they have *very few* listening ears. The point of this is that my fears went away *after* experiencing that none of them came true.

MY FEARS WENT AWAY *AFTER* EXPERIENCING THAT
NONE OF THEM CAME TRUE
- Vera Wilhelmsen, collector of shiny things and self-quoter

If you think a fear is real, of course it won't go away until you *experience* that there was no need for it or that the world doesn't work that way! It's okay to be scared shitless for a while. It's horrible, but you have to hang in there until it gets better! Sometimes you just have to keep rowing until you find calmer waters. It was definitely worth it. All of it. I would never have the freedom or happiness I have now if I hadn't cut contact or faced all of my programmed fears. And do not try to override or "heal" fears that should be there, such as fear of crocodiles, LOL. If you are afraid someone might physically hurt you, then reach out for help and protect yourself properly. I hope this was helpful, and I'll leave you with some methods to try when you feel fear on this level!

- You can try any of these and see what works for you: go outside and RUN for it, like a bear is chasing you! This might help your body to realize more quickly that you are in fact safe and "finish" the trauma, since you have now "escaped." Run on the spot, stamp your feet, shake until you become aware of your physical control over your body, punch pillows, punch into the air, push back into the air like it was your abuser, push into the air with all your force as if you're pushing someone backwards - protecting yourself. Make noises, express things like "leave me alone," "get back," "get the feck away from me, you're crazy," "I'm leaving" and run a little out the door or similar. This feels sooooo goood afterwards. Anything that helps you *feel* that you are an adult, that you are not powerless, that you can stand up for and protect yourself with both your body and your words. Express standing up for yourself into the air or in the mirror. This might help you begin seeing yourself as a powerful being. At least a being that has a body they can use to protect themselves with. Baby steps, baby!

- Suppressed fear also needs to be felt through and processed. Allow yourself to feel it, let yourself feel cold and scared, whatever comes up. Let it be there until it has been digested. In childhood I quickly learned to hold my breath and literally push feelings down with my stomach, such as fear, anger and tears. These feelings never went away, they were stored in my body, and I had to feel through them to release them! It takes time to break through the numbness and get to the feelings, but the more time you spend being aware of your body, the easier it becomes. *Let yourself have the reactions you should have been allowed to have, when whatever is coming up now, happened.* Fall to your knees in despair, lean yourself against the wall while breathing. *React!*

- Dance. Seriously. Try expressing what you are feeling through dance. How does panic look through dance? No one's watching, just do it!

- Allow your fear to express itself. Talk to yourself and say something like "oh my god, og my god, oh my god! I'm freaking out! I don't know why but I'll keep talking until I feel better." See what comes up once you start talking.

May you find peace in your body, again or for the first time. Hugs.

CHAPTER 11

Guilt

GUILT IS ALSO JUST A FEELING THAT CAN BE PROCESSED
WITHOUT BEING ACTED UPON.

-Adriana Bucci, narcissistic abuse recovery expert & friend said something like this. I can't remember it word for word, and she can't either, but it was genius!

The only thing you need to know about guilt is: don't act on it until you've worked through it. I'm talking about the "big" stuff of course. If you're late to an appointment or forgot to cancel an appointment and you didn't show up, then of course simply just apologize. But when there is confusion, if you're suspecting there is something toxic about the person you have supposedly wronged, or if there is especially loud guilt or shame in your stomach, then feel free to pick some advice from this chapter! Use the methods of feeling your feelings and journaling until you are absolutely certain you really have done something wrong. And *then* you can apologize in any way you like, be it a letter, a message, a phone call or in person. You can use all the tips and tricks in this book for guilt as well. Guilt is a feeling like all other feelings, acting on it isn't the only way to make it "go away." It can be processed and worked through. Clarity can be found. I recommend journaling through the guilt for at least an hour before taking any sort of action. There are people in this world who will use guilt trips as a tool for manipulation and abuse. So make sure you aren't feeling unjustified toxic guilt before apologizing or taking action, by working through it. Journaling is especially effective for working through any confusion around guilt!

And if you *do* wish to apologize to someone: *only* take responsibility for what you actually were responsible for. If you are to go down this road then make it something that will give you relief and not leave you once again with that icky feeling of self-abandonment. I used to go a little overboard with my apologies, turning it sour as I apologized for more than I was responsible for. If you take on too much responsibility for the situation then you'll be left with new emotions you have to process, such as bitterness. I'll give you an example: in my time as overly responsible and accommodating to everyone else's feelings, I once made a promise on a whim to make someone feel better. It was not fair to me, but I gave my word without thinking through if this was really healthy. It wasn't. I broke my word. I sent an apology message many years later after working through all the emotional and mental fog around this situation. I apologized for making a promise and not keeping it. I did not apologize for *more* than that. My actions weren't wrong, but making and breaking a promise was. This gives the other person a chance to take responsibility for their part in the situation, if applicable. And your apology needs to be sincere and without accusations or "I did it because." I didn't say anything about my upbringing in my apology, even though my upbringing was the cause of my behavior. I only wrote what I did and that I was sorry. Keep it *real* and keep it *simple*.

A toxic person will usually never acknowledge their toxic behavior. You can confront and say what you need to say for your own sake, but don't be surprised if they'll deflect and somehow make *you* the bad guy. They see accountability and fairness as an *attack*. Please don't listen to deflections such as "I did my *best*," "are you saying I'm a *bad mother?*" "you *made me* do it" etc. First of all, you can't *make* adults do anything. We are all responsible for our behavior, to improve it and heal the reasons behind it whenever necessary. Second, what is your definition of *doing your best*? I would definitely say it means pushing through and searching for solutions until you find one when you're stuck. So ask yourself if the person in question has exhausted all possible options to improve their behavior and become a better partner/mother/father/friend etc. Have they searched the internet for tools? Read books on relevant topics? Gone to therapy? Listened to your pleas? Tried to hold back their toxic words and behaviors? Then you know, they didn't do their best and claiming so is just a tactic of emotional abuse. Getting an apology from a toxic person isn't necessary for your healing. You can still feel relief and closure, just by standing up for yourself and processing your feelings on your own. You can say what you need to say to them in person, in a message or a letter, or in your journal and never show it to them. It is the act of expressing it that is healing, not their response.

Letter writing is an amazing tool for healing when it comes to guilt and any other feeling! You don't have to send the letters, and if you write them with the intention of *not* sending them, it will be easier to express yourself fully and not hold back. If there is someone you can't apologize to because they have passed or you feel like it would be too awkward and upsetting to do it now, then the act of writing the letter will energetically release the situation from your system. If someone hurt you then writing a letter where you don't hold back at all is extremely healing. And you don't have to send it! It's often better if you don't, because if they are particularly toxic they will use the letter to fuel more drama and make themselves the victim. It's up to you. I did send that letter to my toxic grandmother which led to her pretending to faint and my whole family accusing me of "trying to kill a frail old woman." But I don't regret it. I found peace after telling her how I felt about her and her behavior even though she didn't acknowledge it. I realized how powerful I was when I healed and released so much heaviness without needing anything from other people. I was also okay with not getting a reply for my apology to a former friend. Because we can't control other people. We can only work with ourselves.

CHAPTER 12

Nightmares & Waking Up In Emotional Pain

Nightmares. Hnnnnnng. This is a difficult one. I don't know why we have them or where they come from, but through experimenting on myself I have found some methods that might help make your mornings a little bit better and over time reduce the intensity and frequency of the nightmares. I used to have horrible nightmares every night and wake up exhausted and triggered. It *has* gotten better. I still get them, but the nature of the nightmares has evolved from trauma to my current stresses, and sometimes remaining trauma coming up for healing. I realized all my nightmares played out situations that were *socially* the same as my traumas, even though the situations were completely different. I could be flying on an airship through the jungle, but *on* the airship I was excluded and unwanted by a family and kept to myself while they enjoyed their vacation, which I also had a right to enjoy. I think these scenarios played out in my mind so I could wake up and release the emotions behind them. I used the techniques described earlier in this book, especially *validating* and *feeling* as soon as I woke up.

Here are a few different processes I've developed for waking up after nightmares or in emotional pain, they work at different times for me:

- Put words to how you felt in the dream, in your mind, out loud or in a journal. Validate and feel, but not for too long. There's something about the emotional pain in the morning that can last forever, so I don't stay in bed for longer than ten minutes. Get out of bed, as movement helps begin to move the feelings. Then let yourself sob (even if no tears come), retch and burp, or whatever it may be, as you move, shower, or look at yourself in the mirror. Looking at yourself in the mirror while in pain is a profound experience. Just try it! For me it triggers self-compassion and deeper intimacy with myself. Go limp and let the feelings begin to flow through your system. Keep breathing through residue afterwards as you go about your day. Sigh and breathe the emotions out while making breakfast etc. It's okay to feel how you feel.
- Get out of bed, lie down on a mat or on your couch, go as limp as possible to let the emotion move. Retch and convulse if you feel the urge to. Lay there for a maximum of thirty minutes. For me the emotional pain in the morning did not move as well if I stayed still with it. Movement helps me the most. The mind has already been processing all night, so what's left is to validate and release the emotions it has brought to the surface.
- Journaling: Write it down, what you remember from your dream, what you're currently feeling, take a deep breath in and exhale it out. I haven't gotten anywhere with overthinking or overanalyzing nightmares. Allowing the feelings that the nightmare brought up to pass through me has worked out

the best for me without analyzing it too much. If you still feel like shit - lie down, sit with it, or move around with it.

- Gentle stretching or slow movements, think qi gong, or gentle dancing, see what helps the emotion move. Breathe through the emotions, get a hug, hug yourself or get someone to stroke your back. Experiment on yourself!

To summarize: journal first, then feel while being still or moving, or only journaling or only feeling!

If you wake up after a nightmare and you can remember parts of it, then ask yourself what age or age range you were in the nightmare. And what time period and setting in your life does this nightmare remind you of? When did you find yourself in a similar setting as in the dream? When have you previously felt this way? There may be emotions you need to release from around that age/period. Take a journal and get out some pictures of you from that period, see if any emotions or memories get triggered. You can do this later in the day if you don't have time in the morning. Breathe through the emotions and write or say out loud what happened. If someone wronged you then say what you want to say to them out loud, as yourself back then or as your protector now (you can speak as if you are the mother of your younger self or a protector/guardian of them.) Stand up for yourself!

I tried for a long time to stay in bed and feel, using the other techniques described in this book, but what helped me the most was getting up and moving around my apartment, really taking in, and reminding myself of the fact that the nightmare was a blast from the past and that I am free now. Feeling while moving!

What were your mornings like in your childhood? Or in your abusive marriage? Or during a hard time in your life? I feel like my body thinks I am still trapped in my childhood home when I wake up and I need to walk around in my apartment to really *know* deep within my bones that I am safe now. After seeing a couple of rooms it slowly dawns on me that I am now a homeowner in a different city, I live with my amazing boyfriend and I am stepping into my dreams of being an author and a filmmaker! If you wake up with anxiety, numbness or sadness and you feel like you "have no reason to," it's probably a protection mechanism from the past. The criticism and abusive comments used to start right when I woke up every morning, and the fear of the day ahead would always hit me. I knew everything I wanted to do would be sabotaged and there was always an extreme anxiety around anything I planned or wanted. It helps me a lot to get up right away, instead of laying in bed overthinking or scrolling on my phone. Getting up and claiming my day and doing what I want to do feels *good!* I feel my new freedom deeply when I can use the bathroom without anyone being mad and do yoga or gratitude journaling without any interruptions (except for hugs.) I had to reclaim my mornings with the fear-facing techniques earlier mentioned in the "Triggers" chapter, which means I journaled and took it slowly while feeling triggered and uncomfortable, to eventually get used to having beautiful mornings. So if you wake up with anxiety, try to identify what you're afraid of and make a plan to face those fears or reclaim that area of your life!

I recently discovered a tight spot on my cheek, very close to the jaw joint. I pressed it and massaged it and suddenly felt feelings of sadness. This was right before bed. My dreams/nightmares were filled with situations where I was unwanted and a fifth wheel. I knew this feeling all too well growing up and it was so overwhelming that it had lodged itself into my tissues as I was unable to process it at the time. When I woke up I massaged the tight spot some more while allowing myself to feel the pain of being so unwanted, while also reminding myself that I will never have to go through any of those situations again. I don't allow toxic people access to me anymore and I would never chase after anyone who doesn't like me or doesn't value my company. I have become myself and I have magnetic energy now. I held the wounded inner-child-me and showed her our new life where no such bullshit is allowed entrance. I kid you not, I walked through my apartment as if I was taking someone on a tour. And I was! I was taking little Vera on a tour of our new apartment and our new life! She was so happy!

Last but not least, let's talk about *falling asleep*. If I can't sleep because of emotions or fear, then that's what I'm supposed to work on. The inner work and my healing is more important than whatever I've got going on tomorrow anyway. If it takes two hours to process all the fear I'm feeling then so be it. Every time I do healing work I shift my entire life onto a better timeline and trajectory anyway. I get back the time and energy lost in a thousandfold. The things I'm worried about being tired while doing tomorrow might be upgraded to different and better things *because* of the hours spent processing fear instead of sleeping. Internal work is always followed by external upgrades. An example of this is that the inner work led me to being able to write a book and be in film school instead of working an uninspiring job! My life shifted and upgraded because of the time I put into healing myself! My energy levels increased because I processed trauma and I realized I wanted to go to film school because I connected with myself through journaling! And it wasn't like I could have slept anyway because those emotions weren't going away until I worked on them. I journal and/or feel until I eventually fall asleep.

CHAPTER 13

Additional Exercises

Now that you've done a lot of grunt work through journaling and feeling, here are some additional exercises you can try as a cherry on top of your amazing, brave healing journey!

THE GREAT PURGE

I unknowingly began developing this exercise in 2009. I was sixteen years old, suicidal and in the psychiatric care facility for acute cases I mentioned in My Story. I had a journal and no internet, so I started writing. A lot of memories were pushing to come out. I started writing down all the ways I could remember my mom hurting me from birth to my current age. I filled the entire journal! It felt good in the moment, but then I felt insanely guilty and shredded every page. Acknowledging how my mom had hurt me made me feel like a "bad" daughter. Confronting her with her actions, even only by myself, made me feel mean. The level of brainwashing I was under makes me want to barf. It was too early to look at it, because none of the adults would believe me or help me, and I couldn't move out on my own, so there I was with all of this pain staring me in the face - unable to do anything about it. I was terrified someone would find out what I had written down. I couldn't leave "proof" of what a bad daughter I was laying around! I knew deep down that I would have to face this eventually, but since it didn't lead me anywhere to acknowledge pain, truth or emotions - I shoved them back down *hard* and tried the psychiatrist's and my parent's way instead: taking the blame for being a "good girl" and pressing on pretending everything was fine instead. They can all suck my dick. FUCK. YOU. Ten unnecessary, completely avoidable years of suffering later, I found myself staring that same pain in the face once again - but this time I was a legal adult, independent of the opinion of "professionals" and my parents, and I *knew* the answers were inside the black, bruised hole of pain. I had tried *not* going in there and it hadn't worked, so I might as well try.

The exercise goes like this: Every time you remember something shitty that happened to you, or how someone mistreated you, write it down in a document on your computer or in the cloud, so you can add to the list on your phone as well. The reason for not writing this in a journal is so that you can insert more memories as they come up, eventually you will end up with a list in chronological order. This is not to "focus on the negative" but to get *full* clarity. Every time you feel confused or guilty you can look at this. When an abuser tries to get you back under their control, look at this long list of traumas they put you through and give them the middle finger. And you never know, it might become a book one day! Section it off with years or age-ranges, such as 0-5 years old, 5-10, 1st grade, 2nd grade, elementary school, middle school, high school, university - however you want! This isn't an exercise you need to sit down for, just simply write memories down when they randomly appear. Maybe they come up when you're out and about or when you are spending some time feeling your feelings. Memories can come up at *any time*. Let them. And let the feelings come through as well. Take two minutes and write them down even when you're busy!

We are purposefully bringing up all trauma and repressed emotions from every year. Write down the ones on the top of your head first, then see what comes up afterwards. You don't have to force anything or fill out every year. If memories from other years come up then write them down too. The whole point is to empty *everything*, not to do it in perfect order. Just follow the chain of whatever comes up! Our psyches are intelligent and will bring up trauma in the perfect order.

Writing down this *huge* record of traumas helped me feel a sense of justice, because there was a *record* of all the crimes committed. The pain had also been *witnessed*, even though it was only by me. My inner child needed this. It also ensures you will never forget. When we heal, things can begin to feel like they "weren't that bad" because we feel good *now*, and it's important that we remember and honor what we went through.

If there are any especially traumatic events then maybe begin with a different year or do some journaling to get warmed up. If a memory is pressing hard on your mind and won't go away, then start with that. It might not be as hard or overwhelming to process as you fear. You can do this.

It might also be beneficial to return to the specific memories a while after processing other ages and years, as you might realize new things that apply to what you've already processed. Maybe you realized something specific about your self-image later, and when you go back you realize that you felt that way at different ages as well, and when you go back and look at it again you release a little bit more! This doesn't have to be forced, it will happen automatically.

More memories will come up from ages you thought you were done processing, you don't have to look for trauma to heal. All you have to do is open the floodgates and allow the process to unfold. Healing happens in a spiral deeper and deeper, you aren't going in circles and you aren't getting worse, you're just releasing deeper and deeper pain and reaching deeper and deeper understandings. Keep going!

If you have a photo from a certain year, then look at it and see what comes up in your mind and body. If you don't, then just go back in your mind and try to remember that year. Decluttering or going through your belongings might also bring up what needs to be healed. The music you listened to in a certain time period of your life might also trigger something!

Your birth and the first years of your life won't be remembered in the same way as the rest of your memories. But maybe you have *feelings* from that age, then write them down and feel them! Honor them! For me, my mother used to talk about my birth all the time and that felt really bad, so I wrote down the things she told me and how she first made it sound very dramatic for her, and then she would turn around and minimize the danger I was in and how it sounded like she didn't care at all if she had lost me. She made me feel worthless, unimportant and like a nuisance. *Stories* around your birth can also be traumas. Ask yourself these questions and journal what comes up; Was I loved and well cared for when I was carried? How was my birth or my entrance into this family? Was I treasured? What was I told about my birth?

What were your teenage years like? Were you supported as you experimented and found yourself? Me neither, haha. But it is *never* too late for self-discovery! Feel it, grieve it, and get what is yours *now*!

Go down the path and journal out, feel or visualize whatever memories come up. What were you told in that memory? How were you told to see yourself and what happened? Did you take on the blame? Was that fair? Were you even *old enough* to have that kind of responsibility? Reexamine all of this from your perspective *now*. Maybe it *was* that bad and you weren't allowed to process it at the time. Some memories are good to revisit with a therapist or a healthy party as we tend to take on waaaaay too much self-blame. This other party can give us a more objective view on the situation and help us realize what part we played or didn't play. Let all emotions surface. Let the tears come. You are grieving that little child's or the past you's pain. Witnessing, seeing and grieving the pain you had to endure as a child might satisfy a lot of needs, such as the need to be believed and maybe even the need for justice as in my case. You are giving to yourself what you used to seek from others. You are so powerful and no one can hold anything over you when you *give yourself everything*. This is true freedom. I've found myself craving a lot less of being believed and validated by others and I also feel less of a need to tell the world about what was done to me. Because *I* have witnessed, seen, heard, validated and believed *myself* and my inner child and my memories. I don't care who believes me or not anymore, as I know that the right people do and that my story will reach those whom it is meant to help and no one else. If it helps improve mental health care in Norway too, then that will be a *huge* super-fulfilling bonus for me. But if not, that's okay. Some people will undoubtedly say I'm writing this book for attention (probably the people who don't feature well in it, haha), and that's okay. Maybe one day they will do the inner work too. And I *am* a fucking star, so bring on the attention! ;)

CONNECTING ALL PREVIOUS VERSIONS OF YOU

Print or gather one photo from *every* year of your life. It is especially powerful if you choose pictures you think you look ugly in, or pictures that are less flattering. Look at them all and see how they are all you. Send love to the versions of you you aren't proud of. Send extra love to the you's in the years you were in the most pain. Feel and release the emotions that get stirred. The point of this exercise is to see your evolution and to grow to love the previous versions of you. If you don't have childhood photos, or if there are years without photos, then find small trinkets or items that can represent that year for you. Maybe it is a Pokémon card, a small rock (maybe you liked to collect rocks as a child?), a snail shell, a candy wrapper or a small drawing you can draw today and insert between the other photos. Whether you have photos, trinkets or both, find a beautiful box or a photo album to put them in. If you choose box, find or decorate a box that the child version of you would have *loved*. This can be an old lunchbox with Pokémons you find in a thrift store, or a beautiful gift box. I recommend thrift stores, book stores or somewhere they sell gift wrapping, to look for boxes. For myself, I bought a beautiful fuchsia glitter gift box for my photos and trinkets. I now display it on a shelf and I put lots of crystals and seashells on top of it. If you don't want to see it every day then keep it out of sight. Keep the box where you keep sentimental items. I really recommend decluttering with the KonMari process and keeping a few sentimental items in a box that *sparks joy*. For me it felt like the few items I kept from my childhood were transformed when I decluttered them and put what

I chose to keep in a box of my choosing that really felt like me. The heaviness lifted.

Sorting through photos can be a very heavy task, so take your time and take lots of breaks. This exercise might take a year or more. It is completely okay to do it on and off. Take a three-month break if you need to. Go with the emotional flow. Just keep going, keep processing and releasing emotions. It is painful and isn't easy. It's like surgery - it gets worse before it gets better.

Looking at photos of myself has helped improve my feelings of *not being real* or feeling somewhat invisible and not as real and physically solid as other people, which I've struggled with. I also didn't know what my face or my eyes looked like. I couldn't name my eye color even when I looked at photos or in the mirror, as it triggered confusion and brain fog. It was as if there was static around me if I thought about myself or looked at myself. Damn, I was really psychollogically fucked up from the abuse! This is serious shit! But now I am beginning to have a clearer image of what I look like, in my mind! I can now look at myself in the mirror and what looks back now feels more consistent and real. I can now more clearly see my face shape and eye color and I remember my complexion when I buy makeup or clothing. I have also grown to love my hair color, which was not "blonde enough" or "light enough" for my mother. I was always "too dark" and "too warm." I appreciate my dark green eyes, warm skin and golden/red hair! All the processing helped me come back into myself and to feel *real* and beautiful!

CONNECT WITH YOUR INNER CHILD

Imagine your inner child sitting in front of you. How old are they? What do they look like? Imagine stepping into them. Now, feel what they feel and express what they need to express! What do they want to say? And what do they feel like doing? Hiding? Go back and forth between the adult you and the child you in your mind or physically change places in the room. Do not say anything you don't 100% mean because the child you always picks up on inauthenticity. If you can't say you love them and mean it, say something like "It's not your fault I cannot love you as much as you deserve right now. I am working on it and I hope you will have patience with me while I walk the path to meet you where you deserve to be met, where you are loved unconditionally." Say "I love you" at a later time.

My inner child shouted stuff like "you wish you had a different inner child! Someone else! Someone prettier! Not a loser like me! There's something wrong with me, you know! Everyone thinks so, so it must be true!" I am happy to report that my inner child is feeling better, although we still connect and heal from time to time. I started keeping a childhood photo of me on my desk after she revealed this to me, to learn to look at my child-self with love. To check if I *really* was ugly after all as a child and to grow love and a clearer self-image. Try keeping a photo of you as a child somewhere you see it often, and choose a childhood photo that does not trigger you too much. If this is too triggering altogether, then revisit this exercise at a later time.

Give yourself and your inner child a thousand hugs when you feel ready <3

THE GREAT MANTRA

Hare Krishna Hare Krishna
Krishna Krishna Hare Hare
Hare Rama Hare Rama
Rama Rama Hare Hare

This one is a purger, I apologize in advance, haha! This mantra is the "maha mantra" or "the great mantra" in yoga - the mantra of all mantras. You can say it without joining any religion or cult. It is a timeless mantra which anyone can use to cleanse their mind and nervous system and connect back with their soul and God/The Universe (whatever floats your boat.) Ideally we sit down and open our session by saying "Gauranga," then we chant the maha mantra 108 times, and then we end the sessions with "Haribol." "Haribol" means "chant the holy name," you can incorporate it if or when you feel comfortable. "Krishna" is another name for God and so is "Gauranga." You can still receive the benefits of this meditation without embracing the spiritual aspects. BUT, 108 rounds of the maha mantra often takes me more than thirty minutes, especially if deep emotions come up and I have to say it slowly and do some breathing between each mantra, so instead of doing it for 108 times or none at all, I do it for ten minutes or for as long as I feel like doing it. I also sometimes say it three or four times before moving on to journaling or feeling/meditating on my emotions. When the emotions are especially heavy, and breathing, let alone chanting, feels like the heaviest task in the world, you can try holding tones for longer, to sing out your grief, "Haaaaaaaaaaaaaaaaaaareeeeee Kriiiiii-iiiiiiishnaaaaaaaaaaaaaaaaaaaaaaaaa" etc. And take your time between the mantras to breathe through your feelings, sob, retch or whatever happens! It isn't always about the number of mantras, but the depth of the healing! It gets easier and easier to chant a larger number, so don't force it!

When I started doing this, my eyes would start to run and burn, and I would feel extreme upwards pressure in my head. I also felt soreness in my chest after meditation. I think the symptoms were caused by being triggered by the act of meditation (it would not be safe to meditate in my childhood home, my mom would mock me and criticize me) - and the purging itself. So go easy! This exercise might be too forceful in the beginning of your healing journey. I had to take a six month break and do some heavy lifting with journaling and being present with my emotions before I could return. We shouldn't cleanse or heal too fast!

I've found that it is especially good for bringing up feelings of hopelessness, heaviness, grief and fear. It cleanses you of old toxins and fills you up with divine love :) Ride the waves! Remember the tunnel! You're not in a hole, you're in a tunnel! Keep feeling and suddenly you will come out on the other side!

I usually sit instead of lying down when I chant, as it makes it easier to tilt my head back and move emotions up if I need to, but it can also be done while lying down or walking - experiment and find out what works for you at different times! Sometimes I do it in bed if I can't sleep, it calms my mind and purges anything running in circles keeping me from sleeping! Best of luck!

SOURCES

1. Accessed April 11th 2022:
Merriam Webster
https://www.merriam-webster.com/dictionary/narcissistic%20personality%20disorder

Thank you for diving deep within yourself!

Thank you for being brave!

Your ripple effects will change the world

Use these tools or find your own

Let us be the generation that heals ourselves, so that eventually healing work is no longer neccessary

Let us be the last generation in our lineage that experienced trauma

It is time for trauma to die out

After this work, you can do whatever you want

Go!

Go share your gifts!

Go shake things up!

Go f*ck up some sh*t!

Go enjoy yourself!

Go *live!*

- Vera

ACKNOWLEDGEMENTS

Thank you so much, miss Naomi Kyllo Bandeh, for proof-reading my book for free! You did me a solid, girl! It seems I always meet the right people at the right time!

Thank you to my super-tall-dark-and-handsome boyfriend for helping me out of the fog, for being a prime example of patience, safety and love - and for cheering me on in all my endeavors!

Thank you to my best friend Ida, who knew me before I became myself, and who applauded my transformation!

I also need to acknowledge my beautiful cousin Charlotte, whose death almost destroyed me, but eventually helped me build a new perspective on life. I miss you but I also thank you for what you taught me. I think of you every time I dance, laugh, and give zero fucks - and when I go for what I want. Your spirit lives on.

And to my friend Dag, whom I always thought would live life parallelly to me - you are missed and I wish we could have healed together. I know we would have a lot to talk about.

And to everyone we have lost to suicide - I'm sorry you were treated so badly. It wasn't your fault. You have nothing to be ashamed about. It's the people and the systems who mistreated you who should have felt your pain. Your pain did not come from anything faulty within you - they lied to you and convinced you to blame yourself. I will use my voice to honor you.

I'd also like to thank myself for facing my fears and publishing this book - and for being a badass in general.

And I need to thank this book for triggering the FUCK out of me and helping me heal even more. Right before publishing I wanted to scrap everything and live out my days somewhere unknown - until I realized that this came from my deep fear of being misunderstood and attacked. I now release this book into the world, knowing that some will love it and others will not. If toxic healthcare systems come for me, then so be it. What happened to me should not have happened and it's still happening every day. It's time for change. It's time for truth.

I also want to say "hey!" to 13 year old Vera! WE FINALLY WROTE A BOOK!!!! WE DID IT!!!! :) Don't worry about your fucking Norwegian-teachers and the grades they give you. YOU CAN WRITE AND YOU HAVE A LOT TO SAY!

INSTANT RELIEF METHODS

Feel through it:

1. Go limp or get out of the way so your breath, body and emotions can do whatever they want.
2. If memories come up: feel them and validate them
3. Keep at it until you either feel better or have to go on with your day.

Journaling

1. Write down whatever comes up in your mind. If you have no idea what to write try describing the tension in your body or simply write "I don't know what to write", or scribble until something comes up.
2. Write or doodle until you feel relief. It doesn't matter if you write a coherent story, what matters is that the old energy gets processed and released through validation and love.
3. Write until you feel better. You don't have to feel amazing to know you are done, it's enough to feel a little bit lighter or "done" with what you were just writing about.

Some questions you can ask yourself during feeling and journaling:

- Ask yourself "why?" until you get to the bottom of it
- "what was I thinking before I felt this emotion and is that 100% true?"

ALL THE TRICKS

STRETCHES

- EXTENDED PUPPY POSE
- FROG POSE
- RECLINED BUTTERFLY
- THE WHEEL
- COBRA POSE
- THE BANANA: I made this one up. Put a pillow or multiple pillows under your back, lean back so you turn into a banana, opening your stomach, chest and throat.

MASSAGES

- Massage the chakras or any point of tension. Experiment with pounding, rubbing, patting etc.
- Take a shower. Let the flood of water hit the tight spot, or your stomach or chest if you don't know exactly where the emotion is stuck.
- EFT, "Emotional Freedom Technique." Follow along You-Tube tutorials. Simply tap in the middle of your chest if you want to simplify.

MISCELLANEOUS BUT IMPORTANT TIPS

- Make a sound.
  Say aaaaaaaaaaaaaaaaaaaaaaaaaaaaaaaaaaaaaaaaaaaaaa and change the frequency until it hits the spot and reverberates through your emotional tight spots.
- Scream and swear in your car on the highway. Or in the forest. Or into your pillow.
- Shake and dance
- Lay down and put a *crystal* on your third eye, on your forehead between your eyebrows. Or on your chest, or any of the chakra points along your spine. Move the crystal around with the tension.
- Do energy healing on yourself: push up energy from the depths of your stomach, and up along your esophagus until it comes out of your mouth by breathing quickly or clenching and releasing your stomach rapidly.
- Have someone hug you or hug yourself until you feel better

MUSIC

- Imagine yourself in a music video or a movie. Romanticize sitting with your pain to trick yourself into spending some time on it.
- Put on music that *enhances* how you feel
- Put on music from a difficult time in your life

BREATHING

- Take deep or short "pumping" breaths while laying down, sitting, walking or moving until you have released the emotion. Look up BREATH OF FIRE online (yogic breathing.)

WRITING & INNER WORK

- Write letters to the people that hurt you.
- Write letters to the people you have hurt.
- Have a conversation with your inner child. Internally, spoken out loud or written.
- Say to yourself: "it's just trying to move through my system."
- Let memories play out in your mind. Let the emotions come. Be open for new insights and realizations.
- If memories or emotions come up when you can't properly deal with them, try saying to yourself "I see it too! I promise I will fully deal with this when I get home, I won't forget, I promise!". It's okay if you forget, it will be triggered again.
- Look into "parts work" or "internal family systems."

WHAT WAS I JUST THINKING?

- Ask yourself what you were just thinking before you started feeling this way.

TAKING ACTION

- Is this feeling a *current feeling*? Do you need to take action upon something? If you are confused then journal and wait until clarity comes.
- Are you tired or overwhelmed? Try simplifying your schedule.
- Are there any **external** aspects of your life you need to take control over in order to feel safe and happy? Finances, grocery shopping, cooking or showering?

LETTING IT BE: IF NOTHING WORKS, TRY THIS

- *Get on with you*r day, allow the feeling to be there, let it overarch whatever you do.
- Wait and see if you just need to experience a specific situation a certain amount of times until you realize it is now safe and not threatening.
- Some feelings need to overarch our lives for weeks until they let go on their own. Let them hang out with you like a baby koala.
- Check the calendar to see if there's a new moon or full moon coming up in a few days. A lot of emotions come up to be cleared around these days.
- If you can't break through to a point of tension or an emotion - then wait. It is not the right time for this specific one to come up yet.

PASS-OUT-LEVEL-FEAR

- Make noises, express things like "leave me alone," "get back," "get the feck away from me, you're crazy," "I'm leaving" and run a little out the door, push back into the air as if you are protecting yourself.
- *Let yourself have the reactions you should have been allowed to have, when whatever is coming up now, happened.* Fall to your knees in despair, lean yourself against the wall while breathing. *React!*
- Dance. Seriously. Try expressing what you are feeling through dance. How does panic look through dance? No one's watching, just do it!

- Allow your fear to express itself. Talk to yourself and say something like "oh my god, og my god, oh my god! I'm freaking out! I don't know why but I'll keep talking until I feel better." See what comes up once you start talking.

RECOMMENDED READING

The Completion Process: The Practice of Putting Yourself Back Together Again by Teal Swan

Toxic Parents: Overcoming Their Hurtful Legacy and Reclaiming Your Life by Dr Susan Forward Ph.D and Craig Buck

Project 333 and *Soulful Simplicity* by Courtney Carver

Healing from Hidden Abuse: A Journey Through the Stages of Recovery from Psychological Abuse by Shannon Thomas

You're Not Crazy - It's Your Mother by Danu Morrigan

Vera Wilhelmsen is an author from Norway, debuting with *How to Trick Yourself Into Feeling Your Feelings: Even After Decades of Numbness and Trauma*, after dreaming about becoming an author since she was 13 years old! She is passionate about sharing how she overcame abuse and bed bound chronic fatigue syndrome online. Her message is that it is never too late to stand up for yourself, heal and build an authentic life. She is also passionate about filmmaking, travel and making a good caipirinha!

Connect:
www.verawilhelmsen.com
Instagram: @verawilhelmsen
YouTube: Vera Wilhelmsen